B.K.S. IYENGAR

The World's Most Respected Yoga Teacher

The Tree of YOGA

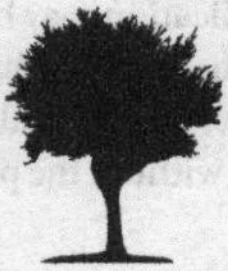

The Definitive Guide to Yoga in Everyday Life

HARPER thorsons

HarperThorsons
An imprint of HarperCollins*Publishers*
77–85 Fulham Palace Road
Hammersmith, London W6 8JB

www.harpercollins.co.uk

HARPER thorsons ™ and HarperThorsons are trademarks of HarperCollins*Publishers* Ltd

First published by Fine Line Books Ltd 1988
This HarperThorsons edition 2013

3 5 7 9 10 8 6 4

A catalogue record for this book is available from the British Library

ISBN 978 0 00 792127 0

Printed and bound in Great Britain by
Clays Ltd, St Ives plc

By the same author

Core of the Yoga Sūtras
Light on Yoga
The Illustrated Light on Yoga
Light on Prāṇāyāma
Light on the Yoga Sūtras of Patañjali

To the yogīs of past and present

Contents

Part Three – Yoga & Health

Part Four – The Self & Its Journey

Part Five – Yoga in the World

Foreword

Friends and fellow-seekers,

In the spiritual world as in the physical world one can climb a mountain from various directions. One way may be long, another short, one winding and difficult, another straightforward and easy, yet by all these paths it is possible to reach the summit. In the search for spiritual knowledge there are many methods, many avenues, many ways to experience the hidden core of our being and direct the mind which is caught up in the web of the pleasures of the world toward the very source of its existence, the ātman or soul.

My subject is yoga – the path which cultures the body and senses, refines the mind, civilises the intelligence, and takes rest in the soul which is the core of our being. It is unfortunate that many people who have not penetrated the depth of yoga think of this spiritual path to self-realisation as being merely a physical discipline, and the practice of haṭha-yoga as nothing but a kind of gymnastics. But yoga is more than physical. It is cellular, mental, intellectual and spiritual – it involves man in his entire being.

For the past thirty-five years I have been coming regularly to Europe and America, giving classes and demonstrations to bring the science of yoga to the people of the West. I regularly give lectures and meet students of yoga who wish to ask me questions and deepen their understanding of the subject. A number of my recent talks and question-and-answer sessions have now been brought together and rearranged in book form, and this book which you have in your hand can serve as a practical and philosophical companion to my earlier books, *Light on Yoga*, *Light on Prāṇāyāma* and *The Art of Yoga*. As you read it, you will discover something of the wealth and profundity of yoga which takes us from the surface of the skin to the depth of the soul. I hope that this volume will be fruitful both for experienced practitioners of yoga and for those who are approaching the subject for the first time. It is my wish to share the joy of life through yoga with you all, so I am very glad to speak to you through this book. Yoga means coming together, and yoga is bringing you and me together through these pages.

Think of the state of mind you were in before you began reading. It was a fresh mind. With no ideas, you came with a fresh mind to look at this book. If we can maintain that state in our daily lives, that is known as integration. To be fully integrated means to integrate oneself totally from the body to the self and also to live in integration with one's neighbours and surroundings.

Integration is meditation and meditation is integration. Those who have no integration cannot speak of meditation, nor can those who have no experience of meditation say what integration is. The two are interconnected and interrelated. If you and I are integrated, the mind is silent in you and the mind is silent in me, yet we are alert and fully aware. If awareness is broken from time to time, that is known as distraction, and to bring the distracted mind again and again to a focal point is concentration. But if this alert state of silence, which normally comes to us only in glimpses, continues for a very long time, that is meditation.

When this uninterrupted awareness of integration of body, mind and soul is retained, then time does not know past and future; time is eternal, and as eternity is here in time, you and I become eternal. That is integration, and in that state no differences can come between us. I hope that if not today, then one day, we may reach this point of culmination. Remember that in self-realisation there is culmination. Probably you have heard something different – that the infinite cannot be seen or reached by the finite. But we have only finite means to know the infinite. When the finite merges in the infinite, everything becomes infinite.

Consider the sky. The sky is finite as well as infinite. None can touch it, yet we are in contact with it at every moment of our lives. Similarly, you and I have to use finite means – body, mind, intelligence and consciousness – to reach the infinite seat of the soul which is the mother of all these things. In this way we remain ever fresh, ever peaceful, and with ever growing intelligence.

God bless you all

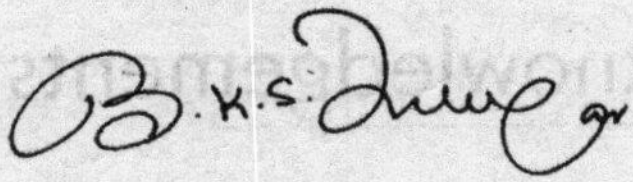

Editor's Note & Acknowledgements

The growing world-wide interest in yoga, and B.K.S. Iyengar's firmly grounded reputation as one of the foremost teachers of the subject, have led to the development of large networks of teachers and students who work under his guidance in many different countries. He himself regularly spends time travelling, lecturing and meeting yoga students and teachers throughout the world. The material presented in this book is largely drawn from recordings and transcripts of such meetings and lectures which took place in England, France, Italy, Spain and Switzerland over the years from 1985 to 1987, as well as a lecture given to the All-India Bharatnatyam Conference in Madras in 1982. Thanks are due to the organisers of these various events for their generosity in making the material available for publication, and also to all those who have been involved in the work of recording and transcribing them.

This source material ranges freely over many different subjects and often moves rapidly from one theme to another in response to the questions and discussion topics that arose. The organisation of this book into chapters and sections bears no direct relation to the structure of the original lectures, and in certain chapters I have included material from many different lectures and discussions where related subjects were covered. Some fresh material has also been incorporated, drawn from my conversations with Mr Iyengar and his own extensive corrections and additions to the typescript. *The Tree of Yoga* is therefore an up-to-date and revised presentation of the subjects covered in the original lectures and discussions. I have endeavoured to keep repetition to a minimum while retaining the freshness of Mr Iyengar's spoken style.

I would like to thank Silva and Mira Mehta of the Iyengar Yoga Institute in London for reading and making corrections to the typescript, Jonathan Katz for checking the Sanskrit transliterations and the definitions in the glossary, Jim Benson for his help in compiling the bibliography and Sheelagh Rivers-Moore for a very helpful suggestion concerning the ordering of the chapters.

The symbolism of the tree of yoga was previously developed by the author in a talk published in Britain in the magazine *Yoga Today*. Articles containing some of the ideas in this book have also appeared in *Yoga Journal* in the USA, *Le Monde Inconnu* in France, *Viniyoga* in Belgium and *Body the Shrine, Yoga thy Light*, published by the B.K.S. Iyengar 60th Birthday Celebration Committee in India in 1978. A short passage in the chapter on prāṇāyāma is reproduced courtesy of *Bharatiya Vidya Bhavan* of Bombay.

Finally, I would like to express my sincere thanks to B.K.S. Iyengar himself for his complete cooperation and encouragement during the preparation of this book, to Faeq Biria for having suggested the project in the first instance and for helping to gather the material, and to all those countless students and enthusiasts of yoga whose interest in the subject makes a book of this kind both possible and necessary.

Daniel Rivers-Moore

Abridged Glossary

A full glossary of Sanskrit words and names appears at the end of this book.

ahiṁsā	non-violence, not merely in the restrictive sense of refraining from killing and from violence, but in the positive and comprehensive sense of love embracing all creation
artha	means, utility, use, advantage, cause, motive; wealth as one of the objects of human pursuit
āsana	posture – the third stage of yoga
ātma, ātman	soul, innermost Self, life principle
bhakti	worship, adoration
bhakti-yoga	the way towards realisation and union of the individual with the Supreme Soul through adoration, and devotion to the divinity
Brahmā	the first deity of the Hindu trinity; the Creator
brahmacharya	celibacy, religious studentship and self-restraint – this is the first of the four stages of life education
Brahman	the Supreme Spirit, the Absolute Being
dhāraṇā	concentration or complete attention – the sixth stage of yoga

dharma	religion, law, merit, righteousness, good works; the essential nature of a thing; the code of conduct that sustains the soul and produces virtue, morality or religious merit – one of the four ends of human existence; that which sustains, upholds and supports
dhyāna	meditation – the seventh stage of yoga
gārhasthya	family life – the second stage of life
haṭha-yoga	the way towards realisation and union of the individual with the Supreme Soul through rigorous discipline and through balancing the solar and lunar energies in the human system
jñāna	knowledge, including sacred knowledge derived from meditation on the higher truths of religion and philosophy
jñāna-yoga	the way towards realisation and union of the individual with the Supreme Soul through knowledge and understanding
karma	action
karma-yoga	the way towards realisation and union of the individual with the Supreme Soul through action
kuṇḍalini	coiled female serpent; the divine cosmic energy symbolised as a coiled serpent which lies dormant at the base of the spinal column
kuṇḍalinī-yoga	the way towards realisation and union of the individual with the Supreme Soul through the awakening of the divine cosmic energy
mokṣa	liberation; emancipation of the soul from recurring births

niyama	self-purification by discipline – the second stage of yoga
prāṇa	breath, respiration, wind, life force, life, vitality, energy, strength, the hidden energy in the atmospheric air
prāṇāyāma	regulation of energy and life force through rhythmic control of breath – the fourth stage of yoga
pratyāhāra	withdrawal and emancipation of the mind from the domination of the senses and sensual objects – the fifth stage of yoga
samādhi	a state in which the aspirant is one with the object of his meditation, the Supreme Spirit governing the universe, and experiences unutterable peace and joy
sannyāsa	detachment from the affairs of this world and attachment to the service of the Lord – this corresponds to the fourth stage of life
Śiva	the third deity of the Hindu trinity; the Destroyer
vānaprastha	the third stage of life, in which one abandons family life for an ascetic life in the forest
Viṣṇu	the second deity of the Hindu trinity; the Preserver
yama	universal moral commandments or ethical disciplines transcending creeds, countries, age and time – the first stage of yoga
yoga	union, communion; the union of our will to the will of God, which enables us to look evenly at life in all its aspects; the method to achieve this

Part One

Yoga & Life

1

Yoga is one

Yoga means union. The union of the individual soul with the Universal Spirit is yoga. But this is too abstract a notion to be easily understood, so for our level of understanding I say that yoga is the union of body with the mind and of mind with the soul.

Ninety per cent of us are suffering in some way, physically, mentally or spiritually. The science of yoga helps us to keep the body as a temple so that it becomes as clean as the soul. The body is lazy, the mind is vibrant and the soul is luminous. Yogic practices develop the body to the level of the vibrant mind so that the body and the mind, having both become vibrant, are drawn towards the light of the soul.

Philosophers, saints and sages tell us that there are various paths by which we can reach the ultimate goal, the sight of the soul. The science of mind is called rāja-yoga, the science of intelligence is jñāna-yoga, the science of duty is karma-yoga, and the science of will is haṭha-yoga. For the authors of the ancient texts, these names were like the keys on a keyboard. The keyboard has many keys but the music is one. Similarly, there are many words by which individuals express their particular ways of approaching yoga and the particular paths through which they reach the culmination of their art, but yoga is one, just as God is one though in different countries people call Him by different names.

Those who approach yoga intellectually say that rāja-yoga is spiritual and haṭha-yoga merely physical. This is a tremendous misconception. As all paths lead towards the source, haṭha-yoga too takes one towards the sight of the soul. How many of those who make this distinction between haṭha-yoga and rāja-yoga have made a thorough study of the *Haṭha Yoga Pradipikā* or other ancient texts on haṭha-yoga? And how many have thoroughly read Patañjali's *Yoga Sūtras*, which are the principal source for rāja-yoga? Do they know that the last chapter of the *Haṭha Yoga Pradīpikā* is called *Samādhi Pada* and speaks of the state of samādhi, or union with the Supreme Spirit? And what is the culmination of rāja-yoga? It is also samādhi. So where is the difference between the two?

If you give a little psychological thought rather than physiological thought to the word 'haṭha', you will learn more of whether haṭha-yoga is physical or spiritual. 'Ha' means sun, which is the sun of your body, that is to say your soul, and 'ṭha' means moon, which is your consciousness. The energy of the sun never fades, whereas the moon fades every month and again from fading comes to fullness. So the sun in all of us, which is our soul, never fades, whereas the mind or consciousness, which draws its energy from the soul, has fluctuations, modulations, moods, ups and downs like the phases of the moon; it is like quicksilver, and as quicksilver cannot be caught by the hand, so we cannot easily catch hold of the mind. Yet when consciousness and the body are brought into union with one another, the energy of consciousness becomes still, and when the energy of consciousness is still, consciousness too is still, and the soul pervades the entire body.

The *Haṭha Yoga Pradīpikā* says that yoga is 'prāṇa-vṛttinirodha' – stilling the fluctuations of the breath. Patañjali's *Yoga Sūtras* say that yoga is 'chitta-vṛtti-nirodha' – stilling the fluctuations of the mind. The mind can go in many directions in a split second. Its movements are very fast and varied. But the breath cannot go in many directions at once. It has only one path: inhalation and exhalation. It can pause for a moment in a state of retention, but it cannot multiply like the mind. According to the *Haṭha Yoga Pradīpikā*, controlling the breath and observing its rhythm brings the consciousness to stillness. Thus, though the *Haṭha Yoga Pradīpikā* begins with the control of prāṇa, breath or energy, and Patañjali's *Yoga Sūtras* begin with the control of consciousness, yet they meet at a certain point and there is ultimately no difference between them. By controlling the breath you are controlling consciousness, and by controlling consciousness you bring rhythm to the breath.

Like camphor becoming one with the flame, the mind gets absorbed in the flame of the soul. This is the culmination of haṭha-yoga. The text tells us that union of the mind with the soul is haṭha-yoga. Rāja-yoga is also the union of the mind with the soul, so there is no difference between the two. Yoga is one.

To practise yoga is thus to unite the body with the mind. For the cultured person it is also to unite the mind with the intelligence and for the still more highly cultured person it is to unite the body, mind and intelligence with the depth of the soul.

Yoga is traditionally divided into eight limbs or aspects, called yama, niyama, āsana, prāṇāyāma, pratyāhāra, dhāraṇā, dhyāna and samādhi. If you are not familiar with these terms, this long list may seem rather daunting at first. In the course of this book, you will gradually become familiar with these concepts and the Sanskrit words will not be a barrier to your understanding.

Yoga can also be seen as having three tiers: external, internal and innermost, or physical, mental and spiritual. Thus the eight limbs of yoga can be divided into three groups. Yama and niyama are the social and individual ethical disciplines; āsana, prāṇāyāma and pratyāhāra lead to the evolution of the individual, to the understanding of the self; dhāraṇā, dhyāna and samādhi are the effects of yoga which bring the experience of the sight of the soul, but they are not as such part of its practice.

Though yoga is often considered in the West to be only physical, it is also a physio-psychological and psycho-spiritual subject. It is a science which liberates one's mind from the bondage of the body and leads it towards the soul. When the mind reaches and merges with the soul, the soul is freed and remains thereafter in peace and beatitude. If a bird is kept in a cage, it has no possibility of movement. The moment the cage is opened, the bird flies out and seizes its freedom. Man attains that same freedom when the mind is released from the bondage of the body and comes to rest on the lap of the soul.

The first level of yoga consists of what can be called dos and don'ts. Niyama tells us what we should do for the good of the individual and society, and yama tells us what to avoid doing because it would be harmful to the individual and to society. These are ethical disciplines which have existed in the human race in all places from time immemorial. Yama and niyama are traditional whether in the civilisations of the East or the West, the North or the South.

Having followed these traditional precepts, or dos and don'ts, we then work for individual development through the interpenetration of body and mind, mind and soul. This second level of yoga is sādhana, or practice, and involves āsana, prāṇāyāma and pratyāhāra. Āsana is the practice of different poses of the body. Prāṇāyāma is the science of breath. Pratyāhāra is either the silencing of the senses and keeping them in their positions passively, or the drawing inward of the senses so that they may dwell on the core of the being.

The third tier of yoga is described by Patañjali in the *Yoga Sūtras* as the wealth of yoga. It is the effect or the fruit of sādhana and consists of dhāraṇā, dhyāna and samādhi. Dhāraṇā is concentration or complete attention. Dhyāna is meditation. Samādhi is the culmination of yoga; it is a state of bliss and union with the Universal Spirit. When you take care of a tree in its growth, in due time it blossoms into flowers and then gives its natural culmination which is the fruit. Likewise the practice of yoga has to culminate sooner or later in the spiritual fragrance of freedom and beatitude. As the essence of the tree is contained in the fruit, so too the essence of your practice is contained in its fruit of freedom, poise, peace and beatitude.

2

The tree of yoga

When you grow a plant you first dig the earth, remove the stones and weeds, and make the ground soft. Then you put the seed into the ground and surround it with the soft earth so carefully that when the seed opens it will not be damaged by the weight of the earth. Finally, you water the seed a little and wait for it to germinate and grow. After one or two days, the seed opens into a seedling and a stem grows from it. Then the stem splits into two branches and produces leaves. It steadily grows into a trunk and produces branches in various directions with many leaves.

Similarly, the tree of the self needs to be taken care of. The sages of old, who experienced the sight of the soul, discovered its seed in yoga. This seed has eight segments which as the tree grows give rise to the eight limbs of yoga.

The root of the tree is yama, which comprises the five principles of ahiṁsā (non-violence), satya (truthfulness), asteya (freedom from avarice), brahmacharya (control of sensual pleasure) and aparigraha (freedom from covetousness and possession beyond one's needs). The observance of yama disciplines the five organs of action which are the arms, the legs, the mouth, the organs of generation, and the organs of excretion. Naturally, the organs of action control the organs of perception and the mind – if one intends to do harm but the organs of action refuse to do it, the harm will not be done. The yogīs therefore begin with control of the organs of action; yama is thus the root of the tree of yoga.

Then comes the trunk, which is compared to the principles of niyama. These are śaucha (cleanliness), santoṣa (contentment), tapas (ardour), svādhyāya (self-study) and Īśvara-praṇidhana (self-surrender). These five principles of niyama control the organs of perception: the eyes, the ears, the nose, the tongue and the skin.

From the trunk of the tree several branches emerge. One grows very long, one grows sideways, one grows zigzag, one grows straight, and so on. These branches are the āsanas, the various postures which bring the physical and the physiological functions of the body into harmony with the psychological pattern of yogic discipline.

From the branches grow the leaves whose interaction with the air supplies energy to the whole tree. The leaves draw in the external air and connect it to the inner parts of the tree. They correspond to prāṇāyāma, the science of breath, which connects the macrocosm with the microcosm and vice versa. Notice how, when inverted, our lungs give a representation of a tree. Through prāṇāyāma, the respiratory and circulatory systems are brought into a harmonious state.

The mastery of āsanas and prāṇāyāma helps the practitioner to detach the mind from the contact of the body, and this leads automatically towards concentration and meditation. The branches of the tree are all covered with bark. Without the protection of the bark, the tree would be eaten away by worms. That covering protects the energy flowing inside the tree between the leaves and the root. The bark thus corresponds to pratyāhāra, which is the inward journey of the senses from the skin towards the core of the being.

The sap of the tree, the juice which carries the energy on this inward journey, is dhāraṇā. Dhāraṇā is concentration – focusing the attention on the core of the being.

The tree's fluid or sap links the very tip of the leaf to the tip of the root. The experience of this unity of the being from the periphery to the core, where the observer and the observed are one, is attained in meditation. When the tree is healthy and the supply of energy is wonderful, then the flowers blossom out of it. Thus dhyāna, meditation, is the flower of the tree of yoga.

Finally, when the flower is transformed into a fruit, this is known as samādhi. As the essence of the tree is in the fruit, so the essence of the practice of yoga is in the freedom, poise, peace and beatitude of samādhi, where the body, the mind and the soul are united and merge with the Universal Spirit.

3

Individual and society

Yoga works on each individual for his or her growth and betterment, physically, mentally, emotionally and spiritually. It is meant for the whole of humanity. That is why it is called sārvabhauma, a universal culture. When you are at one within yourself, yoga does not end there. Having acquired a certain discipline in body, mind, senses, intelligence and consciousness, the yogī has to live in the world without getting involved in his or her actions. This is what is known as skilfulness in action, which does not just mean dexterity. Skilfulness is when one performs one's actions without expecting good or bad results from them. The yogī's actions are performed without vice and virtue, but with purity and divinity.

There is a tremendous balance to be achieved between the philosophical life and the practical life. If you can learn that, then you are a practical philosopher. To philosophise pure philosophy is not a great achievement. Philosophers are dreamers. But we must bring our philosophy into day-to-day life, so that life with its hardships and joys can be informed by philosophy. While being true to our own evolution and development, without giving up our individual spiritual path, can we at the same time live in society successfully? That is practical philosophy.

Yoga is firstly for individual growth, but through individual growth, society and community develop. If a hundred people are practising yoga and can be seen to be healthy, then others will begin to ask what they are doing. In this way the numbers are increased and soon there will be another hundred, or two or three hundred. At one time it seemed that I was the only one who was doing this yoga with zeal and zest, but now look around you, how many people are doing it! So from the individual it goes to the community, and from the community to the society.

Why do you think of the violence of the world? Why don't you think of the violence in you? Each one has to train himself or herself, for without discipline we cannot become free, nor can there be freedom in the world without discipline. Discipline alone brings true freedom. If you have to gain health, do you think you can do so without discipline? Moderation in living is essential. This is why yoga starts with a code of conduct which each individual has to develop. One who is undisciplined is an irreligious person. One who is disciplined is a religious person. Health is religious. Ill-health is irreligious.

Religious life is not to withdraw from the everyday world. On the contrary, we have to harmonise our lives. The circumstances of life are there for our evolution, not for our destruction. The environment will often seem to oppose an individual's life. But can I not live as a virtuous man even if others spend their time in the houses of prostitutes? Or suppose ten people are drinking. I am not a drinker, but those ten people are my friends. When they invite me for a drink, if I say, 'No, I am not interested,' they will laugh at me. So I say, 'I will come. Give me fruit juice, and you take the alcohol.' What does it matter? That means I can understand them. I am with them and not with them. I am within and I am without. That is known as balance. If we can live like that, it is religion.

Individual growth is a must, and yoga develops each individual. But your body is an image of the world around you: it is a big international club. You have three hundred joints – that means there are three hundred club members associated in one body. The blood circulation is ninety-six thousand kilometres long if you take all the arteries, veins, and smaller blood vessels together, and there are sixteen thousand kilometres of biological energy flowing in the nervous system. The surface of your lungs is as big as a tennis court. Your brain has four lobes. Is this not like a big international club in one individual? Yoga provides help to all these parts to coordinate together so that they may work in harmony and concord. Yoga works on your conscience. Yoga works on your consciousness. Yoga works on your intelligence. Yoga works on your senses. Yoga works on your flesh. Yoga works on your organs of perception. Thus, it is known as the global art.

When your body, mind and soul are healthy and harmonious, you will bring health and harmony to those around you and health and harmony to the world – not by withdrawing from the world but by being a healthy living organ of the body of humanity.

4

East and West

It is sometimes said that the Indian body, Indian muscles or Indian anatomy are different from Western ones, and that yoga is not suitable for the people of the West. But is there a British cancer, an Italian cancer and an Indian cancer, or is cancer one? Human sufferings are the same whether one is an Indian or a Westerner; the afflictions of the body are the same; the afflictions of the mind are the same. To call oneself occidental, as if orientals and occidentals were different, is like saying there is an oriental cancer and an occidental cancer. Diseases are common to all human beings, and yoga is given to cure those diseases. Nowhere in the ancient texts is it said that yoga is only to be practised by the Hindus. On the contrary, Patañjali describes yoga as 'sārvabhauma'. 'Bhauma' means the world; 'sarva' means all. Yoga is a universal culture. Just as it works on the whole of the individual, so it is meant for the development of the whole of mankind on the physical, mental, intellectual and spiritual levels. Two thousand five hundred years ago Patañjali did not divide East from West. Why should we do so today?

Then again, people tell me that it is a question of diet – that one cannot practise yoga without being a vegetarian, and that in a Western culture, or a Western climate, that is not possible. This theory is proved wrong as I see that many people in the West have now changed their diet to vegetarianism, as vegetarianism leads to minimum violence. What is more, even the vegetarians in India are as stiff as meat-eating Europeans. Naturally, the cross-legged poses are easy for Indians, but there are many other poses which they cannot do. Do not be deceived into thinking that because they do the lotus pose they are mobile. They only do that because all their lives they sit on the floor, while you spend your whole lives sitting on chairs.

As far as the question of diet is concerned, it all depends what your aims are in practising yoga. Patañjali divides the five aspects of niyama into two groups. On the one hand, śaucha and santoṣa, physical health and happiness of mind. On the other, tapas, svadhyāyā and Īśvara-praṇidhana, burning desire for spiritual development, self-study and surrender to God. The first part of niyama, consisting of śaucha and santoṣa, allows one to enjoy the pleasures of the world and be free from disease. The second part, consisting of tapas, svadhyāyā and Īśvara-praṇidhana, is known as auspicious yoga and enables one to reach the highest state, to be free, to be completely dissociated from the vehicles of the body and to become one with the soul. Patañjali calls these two stages 'bhoga' and 'apavarga' respectively. 'Bhoga' means to have pleasures without disease; 'apavarga' means freedom and beatitude. For health and happiness, according to Patañjali, diet is not very important. But if you are to develop spiritual health, then dieting becomes necessary so that the fluctuations of the mind may be stilled. As you sow, so you reap. Mind is a product of food, so food will have an effect on the mind. Hence, for spiritual practice food is restricted, but not if you are only aiming for health and happiness. It is not a question of East or West; it is a question of the spiritual level on which you wish to work.

I have also been asked whether the individualism on which Western society is based is a hindrance for the practice of yoga. But humanity all over the world is individualistic. How can it be that Western people are individualistic, and not the people of the East? Yoga is meant for individual growth and for physical, emotional, intellectual and spiritual defects to be removed. It is designed for the removal of fluctuations and afflictions, pains and sorrows. Do these afflictions vary from one culture to another? Are they in society or in the individual?

Therefore I say that yoga is universal – it is not given for Indians only. The moment you say that you are an occidental or an oriental, the disease of the Occident or of the Orient is already operating in you. The fundamental disease – that of imagining that you are defective in something – has already set in. So do not introduce these differences between individuals according to what country they are from. Do yoga for the sake of doing it, and enjoy its benefits!

In the second chapter of the *Yoga Sūtras*, Patañjali speaks of avidyā and asmitā, ignorance and pride, which are intellectual defects, rāga and dveṣa, desire and aversion, which are emotional defects, and abhiniveśa, fear of death, which is an instinctive defect (*Yoga Sūtras*, II, 3–9). By culturing the body, the mind and the consciousness, the practitioner conquers the defects of the intellect, brings balance to the emotional seat of the heart, and becomes intuitively strong. Yoga leads to that happiness where one is free from the defects of intelligence, emotions and instincts. The different texts which speak of yoga lay emphasis on different aspects, but all are speaking of the same process of spiritual development.

Do not make distinctions, saying that you are doing a better yoga than this or a worse yoga than that. Yoga is one as the world is one and the people of the world are one. Because you belong to the place called Italy or the place called America, you become an Italian or an American. I belong to India, so I am an Indian, but as human beings there is no difference between us. In yoga, too, some may take one path as a key in order to experience self-realisation while others take another path, but I say that there is absolutely no difference between the various practices of yoga.

In many religious practices one will find meditation and different ways of working with the emotions and desires. You may hear of Zen meditation and think that it is something different from meditation in yoga. But meditation cannot be called Hindu meditation, Zen meditation, or transcendental meditation. Meditation is simply meditation. Remember that the Buddha was born in India and was also a student of yoga. When I was in Tokyo I met lots of Zen masters, and they called me a Zen master too. That means the quality of my work and achievement and the quality of their practice and spiritual development must have been the same. There is absolutely no difference. The essence of the meditation of the yogīs – I do not say the Hindus, but the yogīs – and the meditation of the Zen masters is the same. The Zen masters are yogīs, as we are yogīs. When we speak of yoga, we say it is one of the six philosophies of India. Hence it is linked with the Hindu religion while Zen is linked with Buddhism, so you get differences of opinion and factional disputes. But yoga was given for the human race, not for the Hindus. This is the meaning of sārvabhauma: yoga is a universal culture, not the culture of the Hindus, and meditation is the same.

The rivers which flow in your country and the rivers which flow in my country help to irrigate our lands and make them fertile; then they all flow into the sea and become one single ocean. Likewise, we are all human beings created by God with no differences between us at all. We are all one. The methods of spiritual development are given for the evolution of individuals throughout the world. So do not get carried away by the words which are used in different countries. The essence is the same. Look into the essence and do not be misled by the names.

5

The aims of life

According to Indian tradition, society is divided into four categories or castes known as brahmin (the priesthood), kṣatriya (the warrior caste), vaiśya (the merchant caste) and śūdra (the labourers). Even if today these categories seem to be disappearing as social divisions, they remain present unconsciously and represent different qualities of being which have meaning for us no matter what our profession or place in society may be.

How do these categories apply to the discipline of yoga? A beginner must work hard and sweat in order to learn. This is the quality of the śūdra. When he has become an experienced student, he will express himself by teaching to earn his living through yoga. This is the state of mind of the merchant or trader and so represents the quality of the vaiśya. Then he will enter into competition with his colleagues – maybe he will even teach with feelings of pride and superiority. This reveals the martial character of the kṣatriya. At the final stage, the seeker penetrates deeply into the essence of yoga to draw from it the nectar of spiritual realisation. This is the religious fervour of yoga, and when one acts on the basis of this feeling, one's practice of yoga is that of a brahmin.

These four divisions occur in many other areas. Thus, the life of the human being, considered as a hundred years, is divided into four consecutive twenty-five year periods called āśramas. These are respectively brahmacharya, the phase of general and religious education, gārhasthya, or life in the home, vānaprastha, or preparation for renunciation of family activities, and sannyāsa, or detachment from the affairs of this world and attachment to the service of the Lord.

The sages of ancient times also distinguished four aims of life, or puruṣārthas, and recommended the pursuit of one of the four aims of life during each of the four āśramas. The four aims of life are dharma, the science of ethical, social and moral obligations, artha, the acquisition of worldly goods, kāma, the pleasures of life, and moksa, freedom or felicity.

Without dharma, or respect for moral and social obligations, spiritual achievement is impossible. This is learnt during the first of life's four stages.

Artha, the acquisition of goods, allows one to liberate oneself from dependence on others. It is not a matter of acquiring wealth, but of earning one's living to maintain the body in good health and the mind free from worries. A badly fed body would become a fertile ground for illness and worry and would not be a fit vehicle for spiritual development. Artha is pursued during the second period of life, and it is advised during this phase not only to acquire money, but also to find a partner to lead a family life. This phase allows the experience of love and human happiness and prepares the spirit, through the feeling of universality which develops out of friendship and compassion, for access to divine love. Thus, we should not flee from our educative responsibilities towards our children and those close to us. There is no objection to marriage, nor to the wish to have children – neither is considered to be an obstacle to knowledge of divine love, happiness and union with the Supreme Soul.

Kāma, the third of the puruṣārthas, which traditionally belongs to the third period of life, is enjoyment of life's pleasures, which presupposes a healthy body and a harmonious, balanced mind. Because the body is the dwelling place of man, one should treat it as the temple of the soul. At this stage of life one learns to free oneself from the pleasures of the world and move towards self-realisation.

Finally, to the fourth stage of life belongs mokṣa, which means freedom from slavery to the pleasures of the world. This liberation can only come about, according to Patañjali, in the absence of disease, languor, doubt, negligence, laziness, illusion, lack of will or attention, suffering, despair, bodily agitation, respiratory disturbances and other afflictions. Mokṣa also represents freedom from poverty, ignorance and pride. In this state, one realises that power, pleasure, riches and knowledge do not lead to freedom, and finally disappear. When one reaches this stage, emancipation has taken place and divine beauty shines forth. From self-realisation one moves towards God-realisation. Thus ends the journey of man, who has moved from the quest of the world towards the quest of God, or the Universal Soul.

In the chapters which follow, we shall look at how the practice of yoga relates to the different stages of life's journey.

6

Childhood

The approach of a young child to yoga is very different from that of an adult. Consider the intellectual development of an adult and the intellectual development of a child, and consider the speed of a child in physical action compared with the speed of an adult. Though the child's intellectual development has not reached the level of an adult's, the child sees with universality of mind whereas the adult is more individualistic than universal. Also, the child is much faster in body movement than the adult.

As adults, you have lots of emotional problems. The child has very few emotional problems, and if the child has an emotional problem, it is not of the same nature as yours. If I reprimand you in a class, you will remember till the end of your life that that man from India came and called you stupid. But if you reprimand a child and after half an hour ask what happened, the child will reply, 'I don't know.' Their emotional suffering lasts only for a few seconds, but for you it is lifelong.

Children have speed. They do not like monotony. They love variety and newness in everything. For you, the same pose has to be explained day in and day out and still you do not grasp it. But ask a group of children to do it in two seconds and they will do it very well. A child's mind is in the present and does not go to the past or the future. But adults always move to the past and the future and are never in the present. That is why we have to explain so much for adults, to bring them back to the present. A child learns faster than an adult, through the eyes. If you explain too long, the child goes to sleep, but if I explain or demonstrate fast to a group of adults, they say they cannot understand. Children have to be taught according to their behaviour and adults have to be taught according to their emotional and environmental circumstances. For all these reasons, children and adults have to be taught separately. It is not possible for a young child to attend a yoga course intended for adults. Even if a child is interested in yoga, you will kill that interest if you put them in an adults' class, because they will get bored.

Adults need meditation, but if you ask children to meditate, they go to sleep immediately. For you to go to sleep may take hours, so many of you need sleeping pills, but a child never does. They can be very active, then become very passive in a split second. That is why they get bored if you teach slowly.

I have heard adults speak of children who find it difficult to concentrate. Children concentrate very well. They have no difficulty. It depends on how you attract them towards you. If I speak to children from my mature standpoint, they cannot concentrate on the subject. I have to understand what language they understand, so as to express myself in that language, not in my language or your language. Then they will automatically become concentrated because they are attracted on their own level of understanding. First I must present the subject matter in their terms, so that they can begin to understand. Only then as a teacher can I introduce my new points. Unless I draw the children towards me, I cannot convey anything new.

I will give an example. Some years ago, some school authorities in Pune invited me to teach yoga to a group of ten- to sixteen-year-old children. The school had a reputation as a difficult school. Even now, no teacher wants to teach in that school because the children are notorious and they cannot control them. They asked me whether I could teach, and I accepted.

I knew from the moment I started on the first day, when there was so much noise in the class, that the children thought they could play with me because I was a new teacher. So I allowed them to play with me. If I had been very strict on the first day, the next day when I went to the class I would have found an empty classroom, because the children would have skipped the class and would not have come at all. But when they started making mischief, I said, 'You are very good at making mischief. Come on, a little more!' The moment I said, 'Make a little more noise!' I had won them. If I had told them not to make a noise, it would have been very difficult. That is known as psychology. I studied the psychology of the situation and said, 'Perhaps you should make a little more noise. It's not enough!' That gave them a shock. Then I conducted the class.

Then they were all throwing papers, as children always do, hitting the teacher, hitting a student here and there. So what I did was to observe who played the tricks. I collected together all those pupils, and when I started teaching I called those mischievous boys to come onto the platform and be the monitors of the class. I made them the leaders and said, 'I do the poses. You stand up there and as I conduct the class, you do as I do, so you can be the masters'.

I won the children over, and many teachers from various schools started coming. They wondered how it was that in the yoga class there was no sound. They thought there would be more noise in the yoga class than in other classes because it was an optional subject. Everybody asked how I controlled the children. I said, 'I do not control them. I have not said anything. Sometimes I play with them, that is all.' That is the psychology of children. By coming to their level, physically and mentally, I can then build them up slowly. If I say to them, 'Come on, concentrate!' I don't stand a chance. So I have to be devious, and I say, 'Come on, come on, make a little more noise!' Then I say, 'I love you. I like you because you are very mischievous.' That is how the children come to love the teacher.

Children observe our eyes, so our eyes should be as sharp as theirs. Then concentration comes to them. Children are controlled by their eyes – not by words. You have to give the expression of words through the eyes. That attracts them and then concentration comes.

7

Love and marriage

A pupil who was about to become a father once asked me how a future father should behave towards his wife. This was my reply: 'How can you be a future father? After all, you are a husband before you are a father. You are a husband to your wife, are you not? So you have to behave as a husband – as a true half partner of life with your wife.'

Naturally I know that when they have a child, their love has to be distributed between three instead of two. But no advice is required for this except to live as a true husband, as he was before he became a father, and to maintain that same love and that same affection. After all, what is the child but the product of the love of those two human beings? It is like a flower. So there should be more happiness in the husband and wife to see the flower of their love.

No change needs to take place between a husband and a wife just because a child has come. I am a father of six children. My affection to my wife never faded till her death, and I have not fallen in love with anybody else, though many tried to play with me. As none succeeded, I also advise the future father to see that nobody succeeds in enticing him away from his wife. That is my advice, and the same applies to the wife and future mother.

Now, can you differentiate what is spiritual from what is sensual? When the parents are spiritually united sexually, that first child is a divine child. It is a pure flower of pure love and pure communion. But after the first child, can you maintain the same communion as you had in that first flowering of your love? If that love can be maintained throughout your life, it is a divine love. If the love changes, and if the wife or the husband splashes out on somebody else, like when you splash water, then you must understand whether that is a true spiritual love, or a sensual love. It has to be experienced. It is subjective. Each one can feel whether it is only a sensual pleasure, or a spiritual divine communion of love between two people. Though I have come forty or fifty times to the West, still I have not understood that women say, 'I love my husband,' and then after two or three years, 'Oh, how I hated my husband!', or the husband says, 'I loved my wife, but what happened to that love?' In your countries these problems are very acute, but in India, we seem not to have these problems. When we marry, we live happily till the end of our lives. We do not celebrate the silver or golden wedding anniversary, because we have taken an oath at the time of marriage that we will live by understanding each other throughout our life.

There is a moral concept in the philosophy of yoga which has led to a great deal of misunderstanding. This is the fourth aspect of yama, known as brahmacharya. According to the dictionary, 'brahmacharya' means celibacy, religious study, self-control and chastity. All the treatises on yoga explain that the loss of semen leads to death and its retention to life. Patañjali also emphasises the importance of continence of body, word and mind. He explains that the preservation of semen produces valour and vigour, strength and power, courage and bravery, energy and the elixir of life; hence his injunction to preserve it through a concentrated effort of will. Nevertheless, the philosophy of yoga is not intended only for celibates. Nearly all the yogīs and sages of ancient India were married and had families. The sage Vasiṣṭha, for example, had a hundred children and was nevertheless considered as a brahmachārī because he did not seek only pleasure in sexual relations. Brahmacharya is thus not a negative concept, nor an enforced austerity, nor a prohibition. Actually, the sages who were married would determine by a study of the stars what was an auspicious day to have sexual relations, so that their progeny would be virtuous and spiritually minded. This discipline was considered to be a part of brahmacharya.

According to Śrī Ādi Saṅkarāchārya, a brahmachārī is one who is steeped in the study of sacred Vedic knowledge, who is at all times in contact with the very core of his being, and who therefore perceives the divinity in all persons. The married man or woman can thus practise brahmacharya to the extent that they do not abuse their sexuality, but control it.

Today, in the name of freedom, everyone behaves like a libertine, but the life of a libertine is not true freedom. The five principles of yama constitute social ethics. Each individual should observe a certain discipline within society. Only freedom combined with discipline is true freedom.

For me, brahmacharya is happy married life, since the married man or woman learns to love their partner both with the head and the heart, whereas the so-called brahmachārī, who claims to be celibate, may love nobody but cast a lustful eye on whoever he or she might meet.

8

Family life

People sometimes ask me whether it is possible to practise yoga and lead a normal family life. Is my own example not enough to give you the answer? It becomes personal when I speak in this way, but please do not mistake my meaning. Many swamis and teachers in India and in Europe are protected by wealthy patrons, but I have not been protected by anyone in my life, because I am an ordinary family man. If I wear long flowing robes, I am taken to be a swami, but if I dress like everyone else, I am just Mr Iyengar!

In my early days, many people tried to tempt me to become a sannyāsin. I said, 'No, I will marry. I will see the struggles and the upheavals of the world, and I will practise.' So I am an old soldier. I have six children and still I practise yoga. I have not abandoned my responsibilities towards other people. I can live in life as a witness without being part and parcel of the action. I may be here, I may speak, I may help other people, but I can become completely detached in a split second. That is what yoga has given me. So I am grateful to this immortal art and this immortal philosophy.

Yoga was unknown when I first began teaching. I had to ask people to give me a meal in exchange for a lesson. At times I would practise yoga, drinking only tap-water, without any food for days. When I did get a little money, I used to live on bread and tea, because that was the cheapest nourishment I could get in India in those days. When I married, I did not have any way of looking after my wife. In my heart of hearts I said to myself, 'I am suffering, and now I am making my wife suffer with me.' One of my pupils gave me a kerosene stove, another pupil gave me kerosene, and I bought only one cooking utensil and two plates to eat from. My wife would cook rice and when it was done I would take it on a plate while she used the same utensil to prepare the dāl. That was my life in those early days. Now I have come on from there. I have struggled inch by inch, not only to feed myself, my wife and my children, but at the same time to develop this most misunderstood subject of yoga, which in the 1930s was accorded no value, even in India.

Throughout all the years, and in spite of all my family commitments, I have never stopped doing yoga. I have not stopped for one simple reason, which you could call gratitude. The one thing which has lifted me to the level I am at today is the practice of āsanas. I taught them as a physical exercise in the 1930s, not knowing what I should teach and what I should not teach, but with determination to come up in the world and to bring respect to this little-known and misunderstood art.

I pray to Lord Patañjali, to whom I am indebted for having built me up to this level. I was a dumb student. I didn't even score pass marks at school. I am not even a high school graduate. My education is zero. But from that non-education, yoga has led me to meet people of all walks of life and to discover the world. I learned English only by contact. I continued to practise yoga, but people insisted that I teach. I knew only two things: how to do and how to teach. While practising or teaching, I could express the outer beauty of an āsana with utmost inner attention. Beyond that I knew nothing.

I did not neglect my practice, nor did I neglect my family. The problem with many of us is ambition. You want to perform the āsanas as you see me perform them, but you forget that I have been practising yoga for more than fifty years, whereas you are just beginning. An ambitious or impatient approach will bring you illness – physical illness or mental illness. So treat the practice of yoga as part of your life, allowing it space within your normal activities.

As I have said, there is a culmination in self-realisation. The end goal is the sight of the soul. If one had no end in view, one would not do the work. We can reach the infinite, but we must do so with the finite means at our disposal. Anything done spasmodically has only a spasmodic effect. If you only practise spasmodically, you cannot expect to maintain the sensitivity of intelligence nor the maturity in the effort required to progress towards the ultimate goal. You must cultivate a certain discipline so that you can maintain that creative sensitivity. Instead of working as and when you feel, it is better to work regularly every day in order to maintain the quality of the effects. If your practice is irregular, there will still be some effects, but they will not be of the same quality.

When you have provided a framework of regular practice within the structure of your daily life, you can leave it to the divine force to act in its own time. When divine grace comes, experience it, and go on working. If divine grace does not come today, it may come after twenty years. Even if it never comes, continue to work – at least you have attained health and happiness, and if health and happiness come, that in itself is divine grace.

Do not have it in your mind that you should have something extraordinary to show to other people. If you put a seed in the ground today and say, 'In ten days I want fruit,' does it come? The fruit comes naturally, does it not? When the tree is ready to bear fruit, it comes. Even if you say, 'I want it, I want it!' it does not come any sooner. But when you think that the tree is not going to give you fruit at all, all of a sudden you see the fruit grow. It has to come naturally, not artificially. So work, and let it come or let it not come, but continue your practice. Then, even if you have a family life and family commitments, there are no problems.

If I were a sannyāsin, I might say you should all become sannyāsins and renounce family life to follow a spiritual path. A sannyāsin does not know the householder's life, so it is easy for him to say, 'Leave your family, divorce, and come to me.' These days, many people who are involved in yoga forget their duties towards their children, or towards their husbands or wives. This is not a yogic attitude, but the attitude of a fanatic. The yogīs of ancient India were householders, and reached the zenith of yoga while living amidst household activities, surrounded by families and children. As a family man I say, 'Why should you abandon your family commitments?' You have to find out your own limitations. That is what yoga teaches: first to know your limitations, then to build from them. Then even if you have ten or fifteen children, this need not be an obstacle to your spiritual development.'

9

Old age

It is never too late in life to practise yoga. If it were, then I should have stopped my practice long ago. Why should I do so now? Many Indian yogīs reach a certain point in their lives and say they have reached samādhi, so they don't need to practise any more. But I have not said that up to now. Why not? Learning is a delight, and there are many delights to be obtained through the practice of yoga. But I am not doing it for delight! In the early days delight was the aim, but now it is a by-product. The sensitivity of intelligence which has been developed should not be lost. That is why the practice has to continue.

If you have a knife which you do not use, what happens to it? It gets rusted, does it not? If you want to go on using it, you have to sharpen it regularly. With regular sharpening, you can keep it sharp for ever. Similarly, having experienced samādhi once, how do you know that you are going to remain alert and aware for ever? How can you say that you can maintain it without practice? You may forget, and go back to enjoying your life in the same way as you did before. Can a dancer or concert performer give a fine performance if they have not practised for a year? It is the same for a yogī. Though one may have reached the highest level, the moment one thinks one has reached the goal and that no practice is required, one becomes unstable. In order to maintain stability, practice has to continue. Sensitivity requires stability. It has to be maintained by regular practice.

You may be fifty years old, or sixty years old, and ask yourself whether it is too late in life to take up yoga practice. One part of the mind says, 'I want to go ahead,' and another part of the mind is hesitating. What is that part of the mind which is hesitating? Perhaps it is fear. What produces that fear? The mind is playing three tricks. One part wants to go ahead, one wants to hesitate, and one creates fear. The same mind is causing all three states. The trunk is the same, but the tree has many branches. The mind is the same, but the contents of the mind are contradictory. And your memory also plays tricks, strongly reacting without giving a chance to your intelligence to think.

Why is an old man fond of sex? Why does his age not come to his mind at all? If he sees a young girl, his mind will be wandering, even though he may have no physical capacity. What is the state of his mind? He would like to possess her, would he not? But ask him to do a little yoga, or something to maintain his health. 'Oh, I am very old,' he says! So the mind is the maker and the mind is the destroyer. On one side the mind is making you and on the other side it is destroying you. You must tell the destructive side of the mind to keep quiet – then you will learn.

We are all very good at abusing bad things. Age doesn't count for that, but for a good thing it counts. That always surprises me. I say we should learn to abuse good things! You talk of mind over matter, but in which cases do you apply it? We have to dive right in. Those who understand life and death know this. We are neither swimming nor sinking, but something in between. Life is swimming and death is sinking. If you know these two, then there is no fear. Because we don't want to know them, fear comes. But why should I not face death happily? Fear says that as you get older, diseases and suffering increase. Your mind says you should have done yoga earlier, or you should have continued and not stopped in your youth. Now you say you are very old and perhaps it is too late, so you hesitate. It is better just to start, and when you have started, maintain a regular rhythm of practice.

At a certain age the body does decay, and if you do not do anything, you are not even supplying blood to those areas where it was being supplied before. By performing āsanas we allow the blood to nourish the extremities and the depths of the body, so that the cells remain healthy. But if you say, 'No, I am old,' naturally the blood circulation recedes. If the rains don't come, there is drought and famine, and if you don't do yoga – if you don't irrigate the body – then when you get drought or famine in the body as incurable diseases, you just accept them and prepare to die.

Why should you allow the drought to come when you can irrigate the body? If you could not irrigate it at all, it would be a different matter. But when it is possible to irrigate, you should surely do so. Not to do so allows the offensive forces to increase and the defensive forces to decrease. Disease is an offensive force; inner energy is a defensive force. As we grow, the defensive strength gets less and the offensive strength increases. That is how diseases enter into our system. A body which carries out yogic practice is like a fort which keeps up its defensive strength so that the offensive strength in the form of diseases will not enter into it through the skin. Which do you prefer? Yoga helps to maintain the defensive strength at an optimum level, and that is what is known as health.

Much has been said by certain people about the dangers of yoga, and the risk of injury. But if you walk in the street carelessly, you can have an accident. So do you advise people not to walk? People die when they are in bed. So is it dangerous to sleep on a bed?

I have been doing yoga for over fifty years, and have taught many thousands of students in the five continents of this globe. Sadly, there are teachers of yoga who know very little and claim to teach. The problem comes not from the art of yoga, but from the inexperience of the teachers, and also from the impatience of the pupils. If a person who cannot stand tries to walk, he will break his legs, and so it is in yoga. In Western countries particularly, people want above all to do padmāsana, the lotus pose. They say, 'I think I can do it!' Unfortunately, the thinking is in the head, but the doing is in the knee! If you do not understand the intelligence of the knee and you force it to follow your brain, then the knee will break. But if you understand the stiffness as well as the mobility of the knee, and go step by step to remove the stiffness and increase the range of mobility, then there is no danger at all. If there are accidents in yoga, it is not the fault of yoga, but of the aggressiveness of the pupil who does it.

So you can all do yoga. The Queen of Belgium started doing headbalance at the age of eighty-six. Nothing happened to her. I hope there will be no confusion about what I am saying. You can do it, but do it judiciously, knowing your capacity. If you try to imitate me, naturally you will suffer, because I have been doing it for half a century. You have to wait to reach that level. Yoga cannot be rushed.

10

Death

Death is unimportant to a yogī; he does not mind when he is going to die. What happens after death is immaterial to him. He is only concerned with life – with how he can use his life for the betterment of humanity. Having undergone various types of pain in his life and having acquired a certain mastery over pain, he develops compassion to help society and maintains himself in purity and holiness. The yogī has no interest beyond that.

If we were all at the same level of development, there would be no differences between us in our thinking and in our behaviour. Then the world would have been at peace long, long ago. But we are all in pieces, physically, mentally, morally and spiritually. Hindu thinking recognises the differences of level between individuals. It says we have to accept that we exist from time immemorial, and it is according to our past progress or slowness in development that these differences emerge. A new life is the seed which emerges from the old plant, and it reflects the degree of spiritual development of that plant.

An average individual believes in refinement, in becoming finer and finer. He is like an artist who wants to improve the quality of his life and to be better than he is. The yogī, too, knows that he has to refine himself more and more. He accepts death happily and believes in rebirth as he strives to be finer and finer in his way of thinking and acting. When seeds are sown, the plants come up, and when the plants are mature they give new seeds to sow for the next crop and the next harvest. Thus the yogī develops the quality of his life so that a good seed may emerge, and his next life may bring the harvest of spiritual fragrance.

I have been telling you what my religion says about death and rebirth. Your religion may say something else. My religion says rebirth is possible. We should not laugh at each other's beliefs. Live for the present and know yourself well. The fear of death cannot be overcome by ordinary people, but only by yogīs – and not by ordinary yogīs like you and me! We still have far to go in our practice. You and I are still scratching the surface of the subject.

11

Faith

I am sometimes asked whether it is necessary for a yoga practitioner to believe in God. My reply is very simple: 'If you don't believe in God, do you believe in your own existence? Since you believe in your own existence, that means you want to improve yourself for the betterment of your life. Then do so, and perhaps it may lead you to see the higher light. So there is no need for you to believe in God, but you have to believe in yourself.'

Do you believe in yourself? Do you believe in your existence? Are you here or are you not? Do you believe that you are existing, or do you believe it is just a dream that you are living? This very experience of living wants you to live as a better person than you are. That is the divine spark of faith. From that, all the rest will follow.

There is a tremendous difference between belief and faith. I may believe what Christ has said, but that does not necessarily mean that I follow him. When I was suffering from tuberculosis and got healthy through yoga, I did not believe that yoga was going to cure me. It cured me. That gave me faith. Faith is not belief. It is more than belief. You may believe something and not act on it, but faith is something you experience. You cannot ignore it. If you ignore it, it is not faith. Belief is objective – you may take it or leave it. But faith is subjective – you cannot throw it out.

I hope you understand me when I say that believing in God is secondary. The fact that you are existing is primary, is it not? You are a living example that you are living. And as you are living, you want to improve. You want to be better than you are. This is the golden vitamin which will enable you to progress.

That you are existing yourself, is faith. You do not believe that you are living. Your very existence is faith that you are living. But why are you living? To be a better person. Otherwise, you can just die! Let me see you die! Go and fall in the ocean! Why do you not want to fall? Because you want to live. Why? That is what you must find out. That is faith.

Part Two

The Tree & Its Parts

12

Effort, awareness and joy

When you are practising a pose in yoga, can you find the delicate balance between taking the pose to its maximum extent, and taking it beyond that point so that there is too much effort creating wrong tension in the body?

When you are overstretching somewhere to get the optimum movement, have you ever noticed that you are also giving too little attention to other parts of the body? That disturbs the body and makes it shake. If the root of a tree is weak, the tree itself cannot be strong. Suppose you are doing a head-balance. What happens if you stretch your legs in order to get a good pose and let your neck muscles become loose, or if your elbows do not grip the floor, so the fear comes that you are falling or swaying from side to side? Because the strong muscles try to control the pose, the weak muscles give way. When doing the pose, therefore, you have to maintain a single stretch from the floor to the top without letting any part drop. When you are stretching the legs, you have to send an alarm signal to your arms: 'I am stretching a leg, so don't lose your attention!' That is awareness. Because we lose our awareness and our attention is partial, we don't know whether we are holding the grip or not.

You can lose the benefits of what you are doing because of focusing too much partial attention on trying to perfect the pose. What are you focusing on? You are trying to perfect the pose, but from where to where? That is where things become difficult. Focusing on one point is concentration. Focusing on all points at the same time is meditation. Meditation is centrifugal as well as centripetal. In concentration, you want to focus on one point, and the other points lose their potential. But if you spread the concentration from the extended part to all the other parts of the body, without losing the concentration on the extended part, then you will not lose the inner action or the outer expression of the pose, and that teaches you what meditation is. Concentration has a point of focus; meditation has no points. That is the secret.

In concentration, you are likely to forget some parts of the body as you focus your attention on other parts. That is why you get pain in certain parts of the body. It is because the unattended muscles lose their power and are dropped. But you will not know that you are dropping them, because they are precisely the muscles in which you have momentarily lost your awareness. In yoga there is one thing you should all know: the weakest part is the source of action.

In any yoga pose, two things are required: sense of direction and centre of gravity. Many of us do not think of the sense of direction, yet in each pose, both the sense of direction and the centre of gravity need to be maintained. To maintain the centre of gravity, the muscles all have to be aligned with each other.

If there is an overstretch in certain muscles, the centre of gravity also shifts. Perhaps through insensitivity you are not aware that you are doing this. Insensitivity means that part of the body is dull – that it has no awareness – and this is the part where pain will develop. You may have the impression that there is no pain while you were performing the pose, but the pain comes later. How is it that you didn't feel any pain at the time?

Take the example of a pain in the back at the top of the buttock bone when you have been performing a forward bend such as paśchimottānāsana. If you have this problem, observe next time you perform the pose that one leg will be touching the floor and the other buttock slightly off the floor, and one sacro-iliac muscle will be stretching on the outside while on the other side, the inner part of the muscle stretches. That is due to one muscle being sensitive and the other insensitive. They each move according to their own developed memories and intelligence.

Are you aware of all these things? Perhaps you are not, because you don't meditate in the poses. You do the pose, but you don't reflect in it. You are focusing, trying to do the pose well. You want to do the optimum, but you are doing the optimum only on one side. That is known as concentration, not meditation. You must shift the light of awareness from that side to cover the other side as well; that is what is required for practice.

If you have any kind of problem, you have to observe what is happening in the pose. Is there alignment, or is there nonalignment? Perhaps your liver is extending, but your stomach is contracting, or perhaps it is the other way round. Your teacher can also observe this and touch the relevant part to help you extend the stomach or the liver, so that they are on a par with each other and you find the right adjustment and placement of the physical organs.

In your practice you will find within your own body that one part is violent and another part non-violent. On one side is deliberate violence because the cells are overworking. And on the so-called non-violent side there is non-deliberate violence, because there the cells are dying, like still-born children. I give a touch to the part where the cells are still-born, so that there can be a little germination – so that the cells can have new life. I create life in those cells by this adjustment which I make by touching my pupils. But this creative adjustment is seen by some people as violence, and I am described as a violent or aggressive teacher!

This touch of the teacher on the body is not like the touch of massage. It is more than massage – it is auto-adjustment which massage cannot produce at all. The effect of this touch in yoga is permanent because we make the person understand subjectively the process which is taking place in his or her body. In massage you cannot do this. You use strength and the effect is only momentary. The principle is the same but the effect will not be there.

You should not mix massage with yoga. If you do some good yoga, then take a massage, just see what will happen to you the next day. You will be half dead! Massage is relaxing, but it is forced relaxation, coming from external manipulation. Yoga is extension – extension giving freedom for the body to relax by itself. This is a natural relaxation.

Let us return to the question of effort. If you observe the effort involved in doing the pose as a beginner, and then continue to observe the effort as you make progress, the effort becomes less and less, but the level of performance of the āsana improves. The degree of physical effort decreases and the achievement increases.

As you work, you may experience discomfort because of the inaccuracy of your posture. Then you have to learn and digest it. You have to make an effort of understanding and observation: 'Why am I getting pain at this moment? Why do I not get the pain at another moment or with another movement? What have I to do with this part of my body? What have I to do with that part? How can I get rid of the pain? Why am I feeling this pressure? Why is this side painful? How are the muscles behaving on this side and how are they behaving on the other side?'

You should go on analysing, and by analysis you will come to understand. Analysis in action is required in yoga. Consider again the example of pain after performing paśchimottānāsana. After finishing the pose you experience pain, but the muscles were sending messages while you were in the pose. How is it that you did not feel them then? You have to see what messages come from the fibres, the muscles, the nerves and the skin of the body while you are doing the pose. Then you can learn. It is not good enough to experience today and analyse tomorrow. That way you have no chance.

Analysis and experimentation have to go together, and in tomorrow's practice you have to think again, 'Am I doing the old pose, or is there a new feeling? Can I extend this new feeling a little more? If I cannot extend it, what is missing?'

Analysis in action is the only guide. You proceed by trial and error. As the trials increase, the errors become less. Then doubts become less, and when the doubts lessen, the effort also becomes less. As long as doubts are there, the efforts are more because you go on oscillating, saying, 'Let me try this. Let me try that. Let me do it this way. Let me do it that way.' But when you find the right method, the effort becomes less because the energy which dissipates into various areas is controlled and not dissipated further.

It is true that in analysis you dissipate energy at first. Later you will not. That is why effort will become less. Direction will come, and when you go in the right direction, wisdom begins. When wise action comes, you no longer feel the effort as effort – you feel the effort as joy. In perfection, your experience and expression find balance and concord.

13

The depth of āsana

The body cannot be separated from the mind, nor can the mind be separated from the soul. No-one can define the boundaries between them. In India, āsana was never considered to be a merely physical practice as it is in the West. But even in India nowadays many people are beginning to think in this way because they have picked it up from people in the West whose ideas are reflected back to the East.

When Mahātmā Gandhi died, George Bernard Shaw said that it may be another thousand years before we see another Mahātmā Gandhi on this earth. Mahātmā Gandhi did not practise all the aspects of yoga. He only followed two of its principles – non-violence and truth, yet through these two aspects of yoga, he mastered his own nature and gained independence for India. If a part of yama could make Mahātmā Gandhi so great, so pure, so honest and so divine, should it not be possible to take another limb of yoga – āsana – and through it reach the highest level of spiritual development? Many of you may say that performing an āsana is a physical discipline, but if you speak in this way without knowing the depth of āsana, you have already fallen from the grace of yoga.

In the sections that follow, I shall give a little more detail of what is involved in performing an āsana, and show how within the one discipline of āsana all the eight levels of yoga are involved, from yama and niyama through to samādhi. I deliberately pursue in depth the various levels involved in the performance of āsana, because in the West this practice is too often considered to be only physical.

When we start working on the performance of āsanas, we all begin by just scratching the surface of the pose: our work on the pose is peripheral, and this is known as conative action. The word 'conatus' means an effort or impulse, and conation is the active aspect of mind, including desire and volition. Conative action is simply physical action at its most direct level.

Then, when we are physically doing the pose, all of a sudden the skin, eyes, ears, nose and tongue – all our organs of perception – feel what is happening in the flesh. This is known as cognitive action: the skin cognises, recognises the action of the flesh.

The third stage, which I call communication or communion, is when the mind observes the contact of the cognition of the skin with the conative action of the flesh, and we arrive at mental action in the āsana. At this stage, the mind comes into play and is drawn by the organs of perception towards the organs of action, to see exactly what is happening. The mind acts as a bridge between the muscular movement and the organs of perception, introduces the intellect and connects it to every part of the body – fibres, tissues and cells, right through to the outer pores of the skin. When the mind has come into play, a new thought arises in us. We see with attention and remember the feeling of the action. We feel what is happening in our body and our recollection says, 'What is this that I feel now which I did not feel before?' We discriminate with the mind. The discriminative mind observes and analyses the feeling of the front, the back, the inside and the outside of the body. This stage is known as reflective action.

Finally, when there is a total feeling in the action without any fluctuations in the stretch, then conative action, cognitive action, mental action and reflective action all meet together to form a total awareness from the self to the skin and from the skin to the self. This is spiritual practice in yoga.

The body comprises three tiers, which are themselves composed of several sheaths. The gross body, called the sthūla-śarīra corresponds to the physical or anatomical sheath (annamaya-kośa). The subtle body, or sūkṣma-śarīra, is made up of the physiological sheath (prāṇamaya-kośa), the mental sheath (manomaya-kośa) and the intellectual sheath (vijñānamaya-kośa). The innermost body, on which all the others depend, is known as the causal body, or kāraṇa-śarīra. This is the spiritual sheath of joy (ānandamaya-kośa). When all these sheaths come together in each and every one of our trillions of cells – when there is oneness from the cell to the self, from the physical body to the core of the being – then the pose is a contemplative pose and we have reached the highest state of contemplation in the āsana.

That is known as integration, which Patañjali describes in the third chapter of the *Yoga Sūtras*, and which involves integration of the body (śarīra-saṁyama), integration of the breath (prāṇa-saṁyama), integration of the senses (indriya-saṁyama), integration of the mind (manaḥ-saṁyama), integration of the intelligence or of knowledge (buddhi-saṁyama or jñāna-saṁyama) and, finally, integration of the self with all existence (ātma-saṁyama).

This is how the āsanas have to be performed. It cannot come in a day and it cannot come in years. It is a lifelong process, provided that the practitioner has the yogic vitamins of faith, memory, courage, absorption, and uninterrupted awareness of attention. These are the five vitamins required for the practice of yoga. With these five vitamins you can conquer the five sheaths of the body and become one with the Universal Self.

Since yoga means integration, bringing together, it follows that bringing body and mind together, bringing nature and the seer together, is yoga. Beyond that there is nothing – and everything! In a yogī who is perfect, the potency of nature flows abundantly.

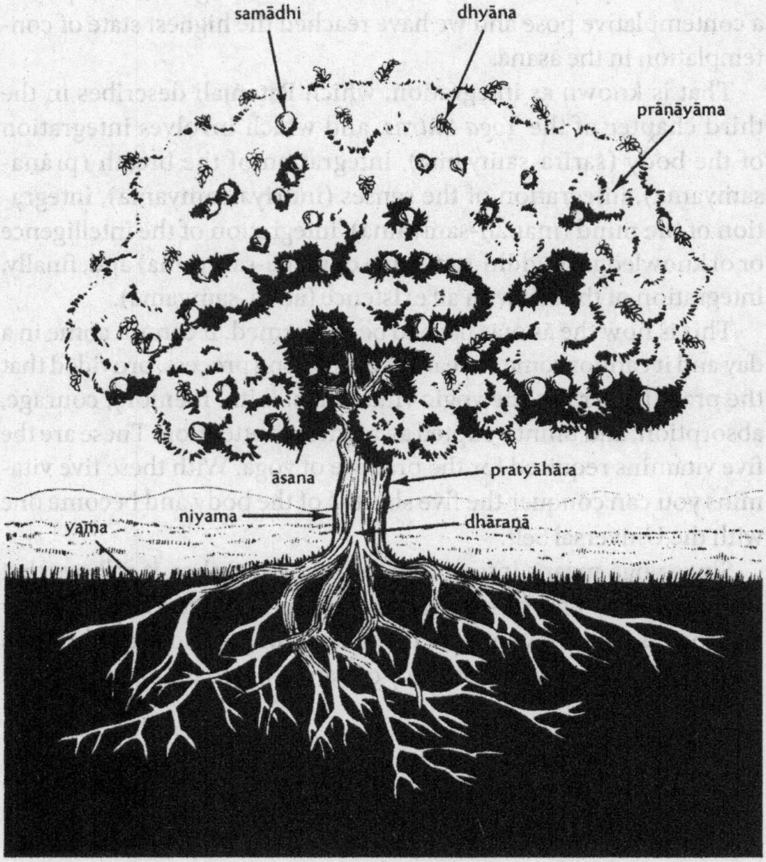

The Tree of Yoga

14

The roots

All the eight limbs of yoga have their place within the practice of āsana. The first limb of yoga is yama, which is likened to the roots of the tree because it is the foundation from which all the rest will grow. Let us look at how the principles of yama are present in the performance of an āsana.

As we have said, yama contains the principles of ahiṁsā, or non-violence, satya, or truthfulness, asteya, or freedom from avarice, brahmacharya, or control of sensual pleasure, and aparigraha, or non-covetousness. Suppose that in performing an āsana you are stretching more on the right side and less on the left. An unethical state is setting into your body. There is violence on the right side where you are stretching more, and the left side, where the stretch is less, appears to be non-violent. On the right side you are being violent because you are saying, 'Do as much as you can! Stretch as much as you can!' It is a deliberate violence because you are overstretching. On the left side, where you are not stretching so much, maybe you have the idea that you are not being violent. But an intelligent practitioner of yoga observes that at the same time as he is consciously doing violence on one side, he is also unconsciously doing violence on the other. Because the right side is more capable and extends further, you are making good use of the body cells on that side, while on the left side you are not making full use of your cells. Though it may appear non-violent, it is also violence as the cells will die when they do not perform their functions as they should. One side thus manifests deliberate violence, and the other side non-deliberate violence.

If you extend the right side more, and if the left side does not stretch so much, should you not observe the duality between the right and the left and make use of the left side intelligently to be on a par with the right? This is known as balancing violence and non-violence, and at that moment both the violence and the non-violence disappear. What is required is integration between the right and left sides of the body, and this balance of the two sides is true non-violence.

When the right and the left are integrated, there is truth, which is the second principle of yama. You need not observe truth – you are already in truth, because you are not escaping by failing to perform on the weaker side. And when there is total stretch in the āsana, there is a tremendous understanding and communication between the five sheaths of the body from the physical towards the spiritual and from the spiritual towards the physical. Thus, there is control of physical sensations, mental fluctuations and intellectual contemplation, and this is brahmacharya. Brahmacharya means the soul moving with your action. When there is oneness of the soul with the motion, that is known as brahmacharya.

Because you are giving total attention to performing equally on the right and the left, there is no attachment or avarice, for when the soul is moving with the intelligence in the body, there is nothing to possess, nothing to seek. There is also freedom from greed, because motivation disappears; when motivation disappears, so does possession, and with non-possession, acquisitiveness also comes to an end.

These are the principles of yama as they appear in the performance of every one of the āsanas. This is what is known as ethical discipline in the performance of āsana.

15

The trunk

The trunk of the tree corresponds to the principles of niyama. What is the role of niyama in the performance of āsana?

The first principle of niyama is śaucha, which means cleanliness. Suppose that in a posture you bend well on the right side of the body. That means you have irrigated and cleansed that side. But if you do not bend the left side in harmony with the right, then your left side will not be cleansed. If you have not irrigated the left side, how can there be śaucha? When both sides bend harmoniously they are properly cleansed and irrigated by the blood, which carries with it the biological energy known as prāṇa.

You know how electricity is produced: water flows like a waterfall onto turbines which rotate under the action of the water to generate the current. So also, when we are performing āsanas, we make the blood fall on every one of our cells like water onto a turbine, to release the hidden energy of our body and bring new light to the cells. When that light comes, we experience santoṣa, contentment, which is the second principle of niyama.

Beyond this contentment, there is a higher state of contentment and a higher level of performance of āsanas, which are expressed in the other three levels of niyama: tapas, svādhyāya and Īśvara-praṇidhana.

What is tapas? Tapas is usually translated as austerity, but its meaning is better expressed as burning desire. It is a burning desire to cleanse every cell of our body and every cell of our senses, so that the senses and the body may be made permanently pure and healthy and leave no room for impurities to enter into our system. It is in this spirit that the āsanas should be performed. This is karma-yoga, the yoga of action, because the burning desire to keep each and every part clean requires us to act.

What of svādhyāya? Sva means self, adhyāya means study. As I said earlier, we are made up of three tiers and five sheaths, ranging from the gross body to the causal body and from the anatomical sheath to the spiritual sheath of bliss. To know the total functioning of these three tiers and five sheaths of the human being is sva-adhyāya, study of the self from the skin of the body to the core of the being. This is known as jñāna-yoga, the yoga of spiritual discernment.

Finally, Īśvara-praṇidhana is bhakti-yoga, the yoga of devotion. When, through your practice, you have reached a higher state of intelligence, and that mature intelligence makes you lose the identity of the self, you become one with God because you surrender yourself to Him. This is Īśvara-praṇidhana, surrender of one's actions and one's will to God. It is the last of the five principles of niyama.

In short, the effect of āsanas is to keep the skin, cells, nerves, arteries and veins, respiratory and circulatory systems, digestive and excretory systems, mind, intelligence and consciousness, all clean and clear. This involves all the aspects of yama and niyama, which are the roots and the trunk of the tree of yoga.

16

The branches

The branches of the tree are the āsanas. What is the right attitude and approach to the performance of an āsana?

You have to become completely and totally absorbed, with devotion, dedication and attention, while performing the pose. There should be honesty in approach and honesty in presentation. When performing a pose, you have to find out whether your body has accepted the challenge of the mind, or whether the mind has accepted the challenge of the body. Are you working from the body to get the factual feeling of the pose, or are you doing the pose because you have read in books that it is going to give such and such an effect? Are you caught in the web of what you have read, searching for the experience of somebody else's written word, or are you working to know with a fresh mind what type of new light is cast on the pose by your own experience while performing it?

In addition to this total honesty, you have to have tremendous faith, courage, determination, awareness and absorption. With these qualities in your mind, your body and your heart, you will do the pose well. The āsana has to enshrine the entire being of the doer with splendour and beauty. This is spiritual practice in physical form.

Āsana means posture, which is the art of positioning the body as a whole with a physical, mental and spiritual attitude. Posture has two aspects, namely posing and reposing. Posing means action. Pose is assuming a fixed position of limbs and body as represented by the particular āsana being performed. Reposing means reflection on the pose. The pose is re-thought and readjusted so that the various limbs and parts of the body are positioned in their places in a proper order and feel rested and soothed, and the mind experiences the tranquillity and calmness of bones, joints, muscles, fibres and cells.

By reflecting on which part of the body is working, which part of the mind is working, and which part of the body has not been penetrated by the mind, we bring the mind to the same extension as the body. As the body is contracted or extended, so the intelligence is contracted or extended to reach every part of the body. This is what is known as reposing; this is sensitivity. When this sensitivity is in touch equally with the body, the mind and the soul, we are in a state of contemplation or meditation which is known as āsana. The dualities between body and mind, mind and soul, are vanquished or destroyed.

The structure of the āsana cannot change, as each āsana is an art in itself. One has to study each āsana arithmetically and geometrically, so that the real shape of the āsana is brought out and expressed in the presentation. The distribution of the weight of the body should be even in the muscles, bones, mind and intelligence. Resistance and movement should be in concord. Though the practitioner is a subject and the āsana an object, the āsana should become the subject and the doer the object, so that sooner or later the doer, the instrument (body) and the āsana become one.

Study the aspect of an āsana. It may be triangular, round, rainbow-shaped or oval, straight or diagonal. Note all these points by observation, and study and act within that field, so that the body may present the āsana in its pristine glory. Like a well-cut diamond, the jewel of the body with its joints, bones and so on, should be cut to fit into the fine framework of the āsana. The whole body is involved in this process, with the senses, mind, intelligence, consciousness and self. One should not adjust the āsana to fit into one's body structure, but mould the body to the requirement of an āsana. Then the āsana will have the right physical, physiological, psychological, intellectual and spiritual bearing.

Patañjali says that when an āsana is correctly performed, the dualities between body and mind, mind and soul, have to vanish. This is known as repose in the pose, reflection in action. When the āsanas are performed in this way, the body cells, which have their own memories and intelligence, are kept healthy. When the health of the cells is maintained through the precise practice of āsanas, the physiological body (prāṇamaya-kośa) becomes healthy and the mind is brought closer to the soul. This is the effect of the āsanas. They should be performed in such a way as to lead the mind from attachment to the body towards the light of the soul so that the practitioner may dwell in the abode of the soul.

17

The leaves

As the leaves aerate the tree and provide nourishment for its healthy growth, so prāṇāyāma feeds and aerates the cells, nerves, organs, intelligence and consciousness of the human system. When we are performing an āsana, we can only extend the body fully if we synchronise the breath with the movement. Prāṇa is energy. Āyāma is creation, distribution and maintenance. Prāṇāyāma is the science of breath, which leads to the creation, distribution and maintenance of vital energy.

Unfortunately, some teachers ask their pupils to hold the breath while performing āsanas. Nowhere in the original texts is it said that one should hold the breath. When we hold the breath, are we attending to the pose, or are we attending to the breath? When we inhale, the brain moves forward like a leaf. When we exhale, it goes backward. When we hold the breath, the brain becomes stiff, so how can we find stillness in the body? Any āsana done on an inhalation will end in merely physical action, whereas an āsana done on an exhalation is vital and organic, and produces physiological action and cellular health. Doing the pose with retention is only muscular – that is the way of practising which I would call physical as opposed to spiritual yoga!

When everything is one – when you reach a state of perfect union between your body, your mind and your soul – then you forget your body, you forget your breath and you forget your intelligence. This does not come in two or three days. It may take fifty or sixty years to experience what I am saying. Till then you can use exhalation as a help, because you are a beginner.

It is true that exhalation can help you to do the pose well for a moment because the body is freed of tension. If your stomach is not well and you are constipated, the doctor gives you a laxative; then after a few motions you feel completely empty and free in your intestines. Similarly, the yogī gives exhalation as a laxative so that the tension in the cells of the body is removed. But if after fifty years you are still doing it like that, then you have made no progress physiologically or mentally. See that in your daily practice there is a progression and a transformation. If I were to do yoga today just as I did it when I began in 1934, then my practice would be like a healthy tree which does not give any fruit, or a healthy woman who cannot bear children. I am not doing that type of yoga. I want my action to bear fruit. The true fruit of yoga is not a material achievement or performance. Yogīs never measure the intake of oxygen. That is not what they are interested in. The yogī's interest is to keep the head and the heart clean through the harmony of breath, and this is achieved through the practice of prāṇāyāma The fruit of your action will tell you whether you are on the right path or not.

There is a very fine story in the Purāṇas which speaks of amṛtamanthana, or nectar-churning, where the nectar of life was drawn out by the churning of the ocean. The demons and the angels were fighting each other for the establishment of dharna, or virtue. The angels followed the policy of virtue, and the demons favoured vice. As the demons were stronger than the angels, vice was increasing in the universe, so the angels approached Brahmā and Śiva who advised them to ask Lord Viṣṇu, the protector, for guidance to establish virtue. Lord Viṣṇu's advice was that they should churn the ocean to bring out from it the elixir of life. As distribution was his concern, they could then leave the rest to him.

Mount Meru was thrown into the ocean to serve as a churning rod, and the king cobra, Ādiśeṣa, was used as a rope to move the mountain. The demons, being stronger, took hold of Ādiśeṣa's head, and the angels held the tail. While they were churning, the mountain sank down into the ocean, so they could not churn at all. So Lord Viṣṇu took the form of Kūrma, the turtle, and went down to the bottom of the ocean to lift the mountain so that they could churn again.

This churning of the mountain is nothing but inhalation and exhalation. Like the mountain churning the ocean, the spine acts as a churning rod for breath in our body. When inhalation and exhalation take place, the spine sends energy flashing forwards, backwards, upwards and downwards to produce the elixir of life, or jīvāmṛta, in our system. Lord Viṣṇu in this story is the same as puruṣa, the soul, in human beings. Viṣṇu, in the form of our innermost self, or ātma, causes us to breathe and thereby draw on the external energies which, at their gross level, contain the nuclear energies of the elixir of life. Thus we grow in health and harmony and increase our span of life by drawing the hidden energy from the ocean of the universal atmosphere.

Philosophically speaking, inhalation is the movement of the self to come into contact with the periphery: the core of being moves with the breath and touches the inner layer of the skin – the extreme frontier of the body. This is the outward, or evolutory process of the soul. Exhalation is the return journey: it is the involutory process, where the body, the cells and the intelligence move inwards to reach their source, the ātma, or the core of the being. This evolutory and involutory process within each individual is prāṇāyāma.

Thus, in each cycle of breath, we have two paths towards understanding the existence of God. They are known as pravṛtti-mārga, the path of creation, and nivṛtti-mārga, the path of renunciation. Pravṛtti-mārga, the outward path of creation, is in inhalation, and nivṛtti-mārga, the inward path of renunciation, is in exhalation. On the basis of this philosophy, the yogīs were trained to reach a balance between these two states. Thus abhyāsa, practice, and vairāgya, renunciation, are brought together in cohesion in the practice of kumbhaka, which is usually translated as retention.

Kumbhaka is retention of breath, intelligence and self, where the lifted Lord – the core of the being – in the inhalation is held by the practitioner as long as he or she can maintain it. This is ātmadhyāna – meditation on the soul. One does not simply hold the breath by physical retention, but holds on to the very self, which was raised up and elated through the inhalation. The moment one lets the self sink, the retention of breath becomes merely physical and mechanical, and is not true kumbhaka at all. In inhalation, as I said before, the self comes to the surface, like Lord Viṣṇu who, after descending to the bottom of the ocean, lifted up the mountain to churn the ocean again. To maintain the stability of the lifted self is true kumbhaka. It is a purely divine state of practice in which inhalation (pūraka), retention (kumbhaka) and exhalation (rechaka), are all involved. In kumbhaka, the self becomes one with the body and the body becomes one with the self. It is the divine union of body and mind in inhalation, exhalation and retention.

If you look at breath in the form of the respiratory system, it is physical. But when the action of the breath on the mind is studied and understood, it becomes spiritual. Prāṇāyāma is the bridge between the physical and the spiritual. Hence prāṇāyāma is the hub of yoga.

18

The bark

When you are thoroughly and totally absorbed in your presentation of the āsana, forgetting neither the flesh nor the senses – when the five organs of action and five organs of perception are all brought into play in their correct function and relationship – that is pratyāhāra. Pratyāhāra is usually translated as withdrawal of the senses. This means drawing the senses from the periphery of the skin towards the core of the being, the soul. The moment the mind becomes silent, the self rests in its abode and the mind dissolves. Similarly, when the muscles and joints are rested in their positions, the body, senses and mind lose their identities and consciousness shines in its purity. This is the meaning of pratyāhāra.

We have seen that Indian thought distinguishes between five sheaths of the body: the anatomical, the physiological, the mental, the intellectual and the spiritual. How is it that we distinguish between the mental and the intellectual body? Why do we divide the mind into two parts which for Western psychology are one and the same? We distinguish between the mind, which gathers information, and the intelligence, which has the power to discriminate right from wrong, and to reason clearly.

Philosophy is not Eastern or Western. Methods are given by philosophers for individual development. You may be a Westerner and I an Easterner, but your weaknesses and my weaknesses, your elation and my elation are the same – no distinctions need to be made between them. If Eastern and Western philosophies appear to be different in approach, you have to remember that Eastern philosophy is very old and Western philosophy much younger. Philosophy in the

West is rationalistic. All things are discussed from the intelligence of the head, and not from the intelligence of the heart. Yet a new distinction is emerging, even in the West. There is now psychology and parapsychology, so a new category has come into existence. True philosophy is the blending of the intelligence of the head and of the heart, as we have been taught, for example, by Buddha, Rāmakṛṣṇa, Śri Rāmānuja and Saint Francis of Assisi.

The intellectual aspect of the mind gathers, collects and accumulates information, but has no power of discrimination. Discrimination is known as pratyāhāra. Pratyāhāra is the culturing and civilising of the senses of perception. In much of our life, memory supersedes intelligence. Memory triggers the mind, and because the mind is triggered by memory, we go for past experiences only. Memory is afraid that it may lose its identity, so before the mind has a chance to call upon the intelligence, memory comes in and says, 'Act! Now! Immediately!' That is known as impulse, which commonly governs our actions. Many people are impulsive. Impulsiveness means acting at once without giving a thought. That is why pratyāhāra, the fifth stage of yoga, has been given to us. You have to make sure that memory gives the right response.

The five organs of perception come into contact with taste, sound, touch, sight and smell, and send their impressions to the mind. Through the mind, they are stored in the well of memory. Memory longs for further experiences and ignites the mind, which by-passes intelligence and directly stimulates the organs of action to go in pursuit of these experiences. Throughout this process, the intelligence tries to measure the advantages and disadvantages so that it may balance the memory, the mind and the organs of perception. But they do not listen to the judicious advice of the intelligence. Because of past experiences of pleasure, they thirst for more and more. Thus, demands and desires increase. The desires tempt the mind for further enjoyment. Through this repetitive enjoyment, the organs of action lose their potency and are no longer capable of exciting the organs of perception or the mind. One continues to hanker for past impressions, but fails to get satisfaction. This breeds the seed of unhappiness. Here, the fifth aspect of yoga, pratyāhāra, enters as a true friend to rescue the unhappy person, so that he or she may find happiness in the delight of the soul.

The mind, which until now had by-passed intelligence, approaches intelligence for guidance. Then intelligence with its discriminative faculty weighs right and wrong, and guides the mind not to depend completely on memory and its impressions. This act of going against the current of memory and mind is pratyāhāra. With the help of intelligence, the senses commence an inner journey and return to their point of origin. This process of weighing one's instincts, thoughts and actions is the practice of renunciation (vairāgya). Detachment from the affairs of the world and attachment towards the soul is pratyāhāra. From now on, energy is conserved and used when necessary without hankering for repetitions. Memory experiences new and fresh impressions, and is subdued, becoming subservient to consciousness. It is consciousness which grasps intelligence (buddhi) and makes it rest at the source of conscience (dharmendriya). Then impulsive nature comes to an end, and intuitive insight flows freely.

Pratyāhāra means not allowing memory to play its favourite trick. Memory is made to remain as if non-existent, so that there is a direct connection between mind and intelligence. This process is not described at all in Western psychology, which does not make the distinction between mind and intelligence. These two parts of the mind are known in Indian philosophy as the fluctuating mind and the still, or stabilised mind. If you have mastered this, then yoga is in your grasp and you will have new knowledge and a new understanding of life.

When an object is held against a flawless crystal, it reflects without refractions. Similarly, when the consciousness is cleansed from the clutches of thought-waves, it becomes highly sensitive, stainless, pure and absolute as the seer. From then on, the consciousness realises that the perceiver, the instrument of perception, and the object to be perceived are the same, and the mind can reflect without refraction or distortion. Patañjali says that at this stage, memory, having reached its ripeness, loses its existence, and the mind, freed from past memories, becomes ever alert, ever fresh and ever wise (*Yoga Sūtras*, I, 43).

19

The sap

To bring the wandering mind to a state of restraint is known as dhāraṇā. Dhāraṇā is concentration, or complete attention. It is the juice which flows within the branches and the trunk of the tree towards the root.

Consider a lake. Does the water touch the banks only on one side and not on the other, or does it touch the banks equally everywhere? When you are performing an āsana, your consciousness, like the waters of a lake, should touch the frontiers of the body everywhere. Where, then, is there room for thoughts to arise? How can there be a thought arising when you are doing a perfect āsana – when your intelligence has spread through your whole body?

It is because you perform the āsana compartmentally that your awareness is interrupted by thought-waves. But if you perform it wholly, with cells, nerves, intelligence, consciousness, and the very self, then perhaps you may experience the āsana differently. Learn to do it as a single unit all at once, maintain that state, and then see whether it is a thoughtful or a thoughtless state, whether there is a space between the thoughtful and the thoughtless state, or whether the thoughtful and the thoughtless states lose their identities.

To be thoughtfully thoughtless is concentration as well as meditation. Absence of thoughts is not forgetfulness. You must run along a single thread like a spider which walks along one strand of its web. There is a single thread for the spider to move along, and for you there will be one single thoughtful state. If you forget the thoughtful state, then that is known negatively as a thoughtless state. But to remain positively and thoughtfully thoughtless is samādhi.

The thoughtful state requires deliberate attention. To remain thoughtless also requires deliberate attention. Hence, there is really no thoughtless state at all, and no thoughtful state either. You do not become empty. You remain full and fully aware. This is dhāraṇā, which leads in time to dhyāna and samādhi, and this is how the āsanas have to be performed.

20

The flower

In the performance of āsanas, two avenues or paths are involved. One is the evolutory, expressive or exhibitive path, taking the self towards the body, towards the pores of the skin, towards the periphery. The other is the involutory, intuitive or inhibitive path, where the vehicles of the body are made to move towards the self. The union of these two paths is the divine marriage of the body with the soul and the soul with the body. It is meditation.

We must learn in our performance of āsanas to express the outer form and beauty of the pose without losing our inner attention. The skin is an organ of perception. It does not act. It receives. All actions are received by the skin, but if your flesh overstretches when you are performing an āsana, the skin loses its sensitivity and sends no message to the brain. In the West, you tend to overdo the stretch. You want to get something. You want to do it quickly. You want to succeed in doing the pose, but you don't feel the reaction. The flesh extends so much that it makes the organ of perception insensitive, and because it has become insensitive, the reflection from the action to the mind is not felt.

Medical science speaks of efferent and afferent nerves. The efferent nerves send messages from the brain to the organs of action for them to act. The afferent nerves send messages from the organs of perception to the brain about what they perceive. The yogīs also speak of these things, but use different words. The efferent nerves are known as fibres of the flesh or nerves of action (karma-nāḍī), and the afferent nerves are called fibres of the skin or nerves of knowledge (jñāna-naḍī). Perfect understanding between the nerves of action and the nerves of knowledge, working together in concord, is yoga. In the practice of yoga there should be a space between the end of the fibre of the flesh and the end of the fibre of the skin – a space between receiving the message from the organs of perception and the message returning to the organs of action. If you do that, that is meditation. Usually we leave no space because we feel we have to act immediately. This is not meditation.

You should know that though the brain is situated in the head, the mind exists in the entire fabric of man. The moment the brain receives a message, it will either immediately send a message of action based on memory, or it will pause to discriminate. The mind and the brain look at the message. You reflect on it. You reason: 'Am I doing this right? Am I doing it wrong? Why have I got this sensation on this side? Why am I getting that sensation there?' That is known as reflection. You reflect on the action produced by the flesh, which is perceived by the skin. You judge what is right and what is wrong. When you judge and make an equal balance everywhere, it is dhyāna – it is contemplation. It is dhyāna in the flesh, dhyāna in the skin, dhyāna in the mind, dhyāna in the intellect. There is no disparity between these four.

You have judged. You have reached a state of balance, so there is oneness. There is awareness through your whole being from the skin to the self and from the self to the skin. Then you know how to see outside and how to see inside. There is fullness inside and fullness outside. But unfortunately, in meditation as it is often practised today, we go in the name of meditation into loneliness and emptiness. Loneliness leads to dejection and emptiness to inertia. Emptiness is not meditation. In sleep you are also empty. If emptiness were meditation, then by sleeping for eight hours every day, we should all become evolved souls. Yet we have not changed at all!

In the *Rāmāyana* epic, we read of the demon king Rāvaṇa of Sri Lanka, who had ten heads. These ten heads symbolise the five karmendriyas, or organs of action, and the five jñānendriyas, or organs of perception. King Rāvaṇa had two brothers, called Kumbhakarṇa and Vibhīṣaṇa. These three demon kings of Sri Lanka represent the three gunas, or qualities of being: sattva, rajas and tamas. Sattva is light. Rajas is dynamism, or hyperactivity. Tamas is inertia, or dullness.

All three brothers meditated, and they attained great powers. Lord Brahmā came before Kumbhakarṇa, the middle brother, to offer him a boon, saying, 'I am pleased with your meditation. Ask, and I will give you what you want.' Kumbhakarṇa was so pleased that he did not know what to ask for, so he asked for nidrā, sleep. Lord Brahmā granted his request and he slept for three hundred and sixty-five days a year. Lord Brahmā said to him, 'If you wake up yourself you are immortal, but if somebody disturbs your sleep your death is certain.'

The eldest brother was Rāvaṇa, who carried away Sītā, the wife of King Rāma. He attained such physical strength through his powerful meditation that he brought Kailāsa, the mountain of Śiva, onto the earth. When Lord Śiva asked him what he wanted, he said, 'I want you,' so that he could carry him. But even when Lord Śiva was in his hands, he could not get out of his mind the beautiful Sītā. Though he also did a tremendous meditation, his infatuation drew him to possess Sītā. In one hand he had Lord Śiva, and in the other he had the lust for somebody's wife. He reached God, yet could not control his senses, and carried Sītā away with him to his kingdom.

The third brother, Vibhīṣaṇa, knowing very well that his eldest brother had made a mistake, pleaded with him to give back Sītā to her husband. 'You have seen Lord Śiva. Why this ordinary woman? Leave her. Give her back to the one to whom she belongs.' But Rāvaṇa did not listen to Vibhīṣaṇa, so the war took place between Rāma and Rāvaṇa, and he was defeated.

The two elder brothers were killed in the war, but Vibhīṣaṇa, the youngest brother, surrendered to Lord Rāma, saying, 'You are a virtuous man. Bless us so that virtue may come back to my kingdom.' Rāma granted Vibhīṣaṇa's wishes. Thus Vibhīṣaṇa's meditation alone was a pure, sattvic meditation. Though all three brothers reached the highest pinnacle of meditation, one remained in a tamasic state, one in a rajasic state, and only one was in a pure sattvic state.

I have given you this story so that you may consider on what level your intelligence is functioning after meditation. Is it tamasic intelligence, rajasic intelligence or sattvic intelligence? Just closing the eyes does not give you what meditation is. Pure meditation is one where all one's vehicles – the organs of perception, the organs of action, the mind, the brain, the intelligence, the consciousness and the conscience – are drawn towards the core of the being without any division in that state. Meditation is a dynamic balance of intellectual and intuitive consciousness.

You may all have practised meditation. I too have practised it. You may be doing meditation sitting in a corner and becoming empty within yourselves with that emptiness which comes also in sleep. I do not do that meditation. I meditate, not sitting in a corner, but in every movement of my life, in every position I perform, in every āsana.

Maybe you have read the *Bhagavad Gītā*; where we are asked to keep the body in a rhythmic, harmonious state without any variations between the right and the left, the front and the back, measuring from the central line of the body which runs from middle of the throat to the middle of the anus. Can I adjust the various parts of my body, as well as my mind and intelligence, to be parallel to that central line? Can I sit like that? It is so simple to read, but how difficult it is to follow!

Do my intelligence and consciousness run parallel in my body without disturbing the banks of my river, the skin? Can I extend my awareness of my self and bring it to each and every part of my body without any variation? This is what I mean by fullness in meditation. I am full in my body. I am alert in my brain. I allow my mind to stretch itself, to diffuse, to cover the various parts of my body. Thus, I learn how to be at one with my body, my brain, my mind, my intelligence, my consciousness and my soul without any divisions at all. That is how I practise. That is why for me there is no difference between āsana and dhyāna. Where dhyāna is, there must be āsana. Where āsana is, there must be dhyāna.

21

The fruit

By studying in depth the performance of āsana, I have shown how, even by performing one āsana, the entire human system can be integrated. Yet we unnecessarily disintegrate yoga, which, by definition, is an integrated subject, when we call it physical yoga, mental yoga, spiritual yoga, jñāna-yoga, bhaktiyoga, kuṇḍalinī-yoga, siddha-yoga, and so on. It is very unfortunate. Why do we demarcate and divide that which unites each individual from the body to the soul?

How many of you really know how to do an āsana? How many of those who say that āsanas are physical know the depth of the way of doing them which I have been describing? You need to rub yourself with words and with works. Put the words to the test of your experience. Do not be carried away by my words or anyone else's words. Rub yourself with each word through work and practice. Rubbing means to experience. Go with it! Find out! You develop original intelligence by rubbing the thought with experience, and that originality is meditation. Using somebody else's words and then saying you are practising yoga is what I call being a carbon copy. It is a borrowed intelligence. Borrowed intelligence cannot become meditation.

I request you to rub yourself with my words and with other people's words, and until they are digested, do not form opinions. Then you will enjoy the bliss which is unalloyed, untainted and free from stains. Experience is real; words are not real. They are somebody else's words, but it is your own experience. So put everything to the test of experience. When stability in experience is sustained and when the feeling of experiences does not waver, it is samādhi.

'Sama' means balanced, in harmony. When the soul, which is the cause of existence, diffuses and harmonises everywhere, that is samādhi. Many people say that samādhi means trance, but trance is not the right word for it. In samādhi you are fully aware. Consciousness diffuses everywhere, through all the sheaths of the body and all its parts. And yet we say that the end of yoga is to forget the body and to forget the mind. As the essence of the tree is hidden in the seed, so the essence of the tree of man is hidden in the seed of the soul. You cannot see the tree in the seed, and you cannot see the self in that innermost seat of the soul. So in the culminating moment, the self too is forgotten, but you forget it by going deep into it. Diffusing the soul into each and every part of the body is samādhi.

There are two kinds of practice in yoga. When you are totally absorbed in it, without the reflection of past impressions, but doing and adjusting from moment to moment towards perfection and precision, it becomes spiritual. If you are oscillating, if your mind is wandering or if there is a difference between yourself, your body, your mind and your thoughts, then it is sensual, though you may be practising yoga and though you may call it spiritual.

You are a beginner in yoga. I too am a beginner from where I left my practice yesterday. I don't bring yesterday's poses to today's practice. I know yesterday's poses, but when I practise today I become a beginner. I don't want yesterday's experience. I want to see what new understanding may come in addition to what I had felt up to now. In this quest, my body is my bow, my intelligence is my arrow, and my target is my self. I am aware inside and I am aware outside. We must learn to stretch the bow well before we can hit the target, so go on extending the bow of your body. Then the arrow of your intelligence will become sharp, and when you release the arrow, it will hit the target, which is your soul. Don't worry about the target. When the bow is stretched well and the arrow is sharp, you will hit it.

What is your state of mind when you are practising yoga? For what purpose are you doing it? Is it to improve your presentation of yourself in order to be more attractive to people as you walk down the street? Or are you doing it to cultivate your self from the body to the soul? If this latter thought is there, then it becomes spiritual.

Sensuality and spirituality are like two sides of a coin – if you turn the coin one way it is spiritual; the other way it is sensual.

It is a subjective matter. You do not require a certificate from an outsider to tell you whether your sādhana, your practice of yoga, is spiritual or sensual. Only the practitioner can test for himself or herself whether their practice is divine or non-divine, because the spiritual is subjective, as the core of the being is subjective. Outsiders cannot see the core of the being. They can only see the body and its manifestations. They cannot see the intuitive side. We need not be disturbed by the views of outsiders who look on our cover, the body, and try to tell us whether we are divine or non-divine.

When you get up early in the morning, have you ever noticed the state of your mind? And have you ever noticed the state you are in when you go to bed at night, before you go to sleep, when you are very near the bed and you go to lie down. Can you explain what that state is? Do you think of the body? Do you think of the mind at that moment? Or does the very core of the being go to lie on the bed? It is the feeling of a split second. It is a moment. I am asking about that moment. The bed is there. You are here. Everything is ready, and you just lie down.

What is your state before you put your head on the pillow? At that time you are not aware of the body or of the mind, but you just lie on the bed. And what is your state after you put your head on the pillow? At that moment you say, 'Oh, thank God!', and you have come into your mind. In the previous moment your body was active, your mind was active, your intelligence was active, but they were all drawn towards the self in order for the self to lie down. That is called being in the moment, because there was no presence of mind or of body, only the presence of the self. If you catch that state and increase it in your active life, you can do anything in the world without losing the inner spiritual contact. Contact with your self is known as spiritual or divine contact. Hence you remain divine, though you are engaged with the activities of the world.

When you see something beautiful, does the body see or does the mind see? What is it that sees? For a moment, you just remain there, open-mouthed. You are in a spiritual state. Then you say, 'I see it!', and in that moment you have brought it to your mind. You have covered your self and you have come to the mind.

As I said, it is like the two sides of a coin. If you turn it like this, it is self; if you turn it like that, it is the body and the mind and the world around you. This way it is a spiritual pleasure; that way it is a sensual pleasure. Remember that no outsider can tell you if your practice is spiritual or physical sādhana. I may be meditating, but in my heart of hearts I may be thinking of a beautiful girl. For others, I may be meditating, but inside, what am I doing?

You have to learn to catch those states. Before going to bed, how is it that your mind does not work? When you see a beautiful blue sky, before you say, 'the blue sky', what is the state of your mind? Or when the sun on the western horizon is completely red like an apple, so beautiful that you can't speak, what is your state at that moment? In the lake you see a fish. Something attracts you. But then you cry, 'Look, look!', and you lose your spirituality because you come to your senses.

So you have to be watchful second by second in order to know what is spiritual and what is non-spiritual. I cannot demarcate. Those who demarcate are dishonest. You should learn to see only purification, not demarcation. If my self exists in all my cells, how can I say the existence of the cell is physical? The self exists in the cell. I exist here. If I exist here, how can I say it is a physical body? When the mind and the thought-waves dissolve in a new approach, as long as you remain in that new approach, that is spiritual. The moment you memorise it, it is sensual.

To try to repeat an experience is mechanical sādhana, not spiritual. You have to keep the experience in your pocket, as it were, and then see what is coming today. You should not call back yesterday's experience. That experience has become finite, because it is recognised. Keeping that recognition in your pocket, see what is coming in today's practice. If you work like that, your practice is spiritual sādhana. But if you want to repeat today the experience of what was new yesterday, it is repetition; it is not sādhana – it cannot be spiritual.

A tree has millions and millions of leaves. Each leaf is different, yet they are all part of the same tree. You also have numberless leaves in your various thought-waves, actions, reactions, fluctuations, feelings, failings and restraints, but they are all connected to the same root, the core of the being. You should aim to see yourself in totality, to see the tree in totality without naming it as flower, fruit, leaf or bark. The moment you see the leaf, you forget the tree. Similarly, if you say that you want to meditate and you forget the other limbs of yoga, you are no longer seeing the whole tree.

If you touch a live electric wire, you get a shock. In your body, your intelligence should be like a live wire, so the moment there is some wandering of the attention or some forgetfulness, the shock will tell you that something is running away in your head. This is action in meditation. This is meditation in action. Thus, there is no difference between action and meditation, as there is no difference between haṭha-yoga and rāja-yoga. 'Haṭha' means the will-power of intelligence, and rāja is the soul. Intelligence, being the bridge between the soul and the body, is the thread used to weave the body and soul into a divine union, a divine marriage, known as samādhi, or absoluteness in oneself. This is the fruit of the tree of yoga.

One has to plough the ground to make the soil soft, remove weeds, water and manure the growing plant, then delicately tend and nurture it so that the tree will grow in health and strength and yield its delicious fruit. We know that the spiritual essence of the tree is concentrated in the juice of its fruit, which is the culmination of the growth of the tree. We pluck the fruit and savour its taste. The joy of that taste can be felt, but cannot be expressed in words.

In the same way, the tree of yoga needs to be carefully followed through its various stages if we are to experience its results. Yama cultivates the organs of action so that they may act for the right ends; niyama civilises the senses and organs of perception; āsanas irrigate each and every cell of the human body and nourish it through copious blood supply; prāṇāyāma channels the energy; pratyāhāra controls the mind and cleanses it of all its impurities; dhāraṇā clears the veil that covers the intelligence, and sharpens it to grow sensitive as it acts as a bridge between the mind and the inner consciousness; dhyāna integrates intelligence, and in samādhi the rivers of intelligence and consciousness flow together and merge in the sea of the soul, so that the soul may shine in its own glory.

Thus, the tree of yoga – yoga-vṛkṣa – leads us by its practice through layer after layer of our being, till we come to live and experience the ambrosia of the fruit of yoga, which is the sight of the soul.

Part Three

Yoga & Health

22

Health as wholeness

The word 'holistic' is very fashionable nowadays, and one often hears people speak of holistic medicine. The word 'holistic' contains the word 'whole', which is the true meaning of 'healthy'. When there is wholeness of body, mind and self, this wholeness becomes holy. Holy means divine, and without divinity you cannot truly speak of holistic practice or of holistic medicine.

When a person connects the soul to the skin and the skin to the soul, when there is a tremendous communion between the cells of the body and the cells of the soul, then that is holistic or integrated practice, because the whole of the human system has been integrated into a single unit in which body, mind, intelligence, consciousness and soul come together.

Though tremendous advances have been made by science, medicine and psychology over many centuries, no-one can define a frontier between body and mind or between mind and soul. They cannot be separated. They are intermingled, interconnected, united. Where there is mind, there is body; where there is body, there is soul; where there is soul, there is mind. Yet our everyday experience is of a great separation between these three. When we are engaged in mental activity, we are no longer aware of the body. When we are involved with the body, we lose sight of the soul.

Yoga is a way to move towards integration, but where does our initial state of disintegration come from? It comes from the afflictions of life: lack of knowledge, lack of understanding, pride, attachment, hatred, malice, jealousy. These are the causes which afflict us and bring physical, mental and spiritual diseases.

It is said that Patañjali gave us grammar to use right words, medicine to keep the body healthy, and yoga to keep the mind in poise and peace. At the very beginning of the *Yoga Sūtras*, he tells us, 'Still your mind!' This is like an electric shock which he gives by his words to our brain. He gives a shock treatment to the brain and the mind, so that we may be shaken into trying to understand what is meant. Why has he used these words? If the mind needs to be stilled, it is because it is in a state of fluctuation. But why do fluctuations come into the mind? What causes the mind to fluctuate? Patañjali goes on to analyse the causes of the disturbances of the mind and the lack of equilibrium in the body.

In the *Purāṇas* we can read the story of Patañjali's birth. His mother, Goṇikā, was an unmarried tapasvinī and a yoginī. Having gained tremendous knowledge and great wisdom, and not finding one right pupil to whom to give her knowledge, she prayed to the sun god and as an oblation took water in her hand, saying, 'This knowledge has come through you, so let me give it back to you.' At that moment she opened her eyes and saw something move in her hand. This was Patañjali. 'Pāta' means fallen; 'añjali' signifies the time of prayer. Patañjali was the name given to him by Goṇikā, his mother, because of the manner of his birth. It was he who wrote the *Mahābhāṣya*, the great treatise on grammar. He also learned dance, and through dance movements came to know the various functions of the body, so he wrote a treatise on health and medicine. When he had written these two treatises, he felt that his work was still incomplete, as he had not touched on consciousness. So he said to himself, 'Now let me speak of consciousness,' and began to write his *Yoga Sūtras*, which begin with the statement, 'Yogaḥ chittavṛtti nirodhah.': restraint of the movements of consciousness is yoga (*Yoga Sūtras*, I, 2).

The *Mahābhāṣya*, Patañjali's treatise on grammar, still survives today, as do his *Yoga Sūtras*. Many think that the famous *Charaka Saṁhitā*, a treatise on āyurvedic medicine, was written by Patañjali and that Charaka was his pen-name, but others say that Patañjali had no knowledge of medicine. It is also held by some that Patañjali, author of the *Mahābhāṣya*, was not the same person as Patañjali the author of the *Yoga Sūtras*. But we know that in modern times a great soul such as Śrī Aurobindo could write hundreds of poems every day, and that his tremendous capacity increased when he did yoga, so it need not surprise us that Patañjali, who was a great integrated soul in his own day, could write major treatises on grammar, medicine and yoga, though all three are very complex and difficult subjects. I therefore salute Patañjali, who brought us knowledge and understanding in these three fields.

The *Yoga Sūtras* begin with the very root of the mind and the intelligence, which is consciousness, or chitta. In the first chapter, called *Samādhi Pada*, Patañjali analyses the movements and behaviour of the mind. In the second chapter, called *Sādhana Pada*, the chapter on practice, he goes on to speak of kleśas, the afflictions of the body which cause the movements of the mind or behavioural patterns of each individual.

In the third chapter, called *Vibhūti Pada*, the chapter on attainments, Patañjali describes the results of yoga and states what effects, properties, or gifts can be gained through the practice of yoga. But he warns that we should not be caught out by these effects, thinking that with them our spiritual journey has reached its goal. Rather, we should continue our practice so that the intelligence of the consciousness and the intelligence of the soul may become equally balanced. When they are equally balanced, we reach the highest state of wisdom where the person exists in complete integration. This state is known as kaivalya, and Patañjali's fourth chapter is called *Kaivalya Pada*, the chapter on absolute liberation.

Thus, the *Yoga Sūtras* speak of the mind in the first chapter and of the body in the second chapter, and they remind us in the third and fourth chapters that our final aim in yoga must be to arrive at the soul. Patañjali applied his wisdom primarily to speech in his treatise on grammar, the body in his treatise on medicine, and the soul in his treatise on yoga. Yet within the science of yoga, the three levels of being – body, mind and soul – are all involved. Thus yoga is an integrated science which can lead man's divided being back to wholeness and health.

23

The aim and the by-product

In the first instance, yoga is not a therapeutic science at all. Yoga is a science for liberating the soul by bringing the consciousness, the mind and the body to a state of integration. But when a factory is constructed to produce a certain product for marketing, fortunately or unfortunately many other products may incidentally be produced, and may also have market value. So it is possible to forget the original purpose for which the factory was built, and produce only the by-products to sell on the market. Similarly, yoga has several facets, and though the aim and culmination of yoga is the sight of the soul, it has lots of beneficial side-effects, among which are health, happiness, peace and poise. As every industrial process has certain by-products, so health; happiness and healing are all by- products of yoga, and yoga can to some extent be seen as a medical science.

Our health and our very existence depend on the respiratory and circulatory functions. These are the two gates to the kingdom of the human system, and if either of them is blocked, disturbed or locked, then diseases will result. Suppose that the room you are in is a human body. If the windows and doors are closed, you get a bad smell in the room. That bad smell is the disease of the room, so what do you do? You open the doors and windows, and the bad air in the room is pushed out by the fresh air. In the same way, the practice of āsanas supplies energy and circulation to the human body. When you perform the āsanas, wherever there are impediments in the body due to lack of circulation, so that you are suffering from rheumatoid arthritis, asthma, bronchitis, liver pain, stomach pain, intestinal pain and so on, the postures irrigate the system, and the impediments are washed away. Then, being cleansed of the afflictions which brought disintegration, you come back to integration and life, and health begins to blossom. Similarly, if the respiratory gate is blocked or disturbed, the practice of prāṇāyāma will cleanse the system and bring it back to a state of wholeness.

Āsanas and prāṇāyāma are the fountain and source for all the other aspects of yoga, because the whole human system is dependent on the respiratory and circulatory gates. The regulation of breath keeps the respiratory gate clean and open, and through an unobstructed, undisturbed circulatory system, the blood will feed each and every part of our body. By allowing the blood to circulate to the areas of the body which are unhealthy, they are nourished, toxins are dissolved and the various ailments and symptoms of physical diseases can come to an end. This may take place over a long period of time. It is a natural process and operates at the rhythm of natural processes. Remember that even if you take drugs as recommended by modern medicine, the drugs activate certain processes so that the functions of nature take place faster, but they are not the cure – they just accelerate the process. The drugs do not cure the disease. Nature alone cures the disease. Yoga, on the other hand, uses no external drugs to accelerate the process. You have to depend on your own nature, and through nature alone enable the human system to function as rapidly and as effectively as it can. Therefore it is slow but certain, whereas modern medicine is fast but may not be certain!

According to the Indian medical science of āyurveda, the various physical ailments are due to the imbalance of the five elements in our body. We shall say more about this in the next chapter. The practice of āsanas can bring about a balance between these elements, and prāṇāyāma accelerates the process. I said above that drugs can accelerate a healing process, but are not themselves the cure. Similarly, prāṇāyāma does not bring the balance, but it accelerates the process so that the poses can bring the balance sooner. What poses should be done, and what poses should be avoided, has to be learnt by working with a competent teacher. Āsanas are not prescriptions; they are descriptions. Prescribing means writing out the details of the remedy and letting the patient go and buy it at the pharmacy.

But in yoga, you have to describe the pose and how it has to be done for such and such a problem, and the person who is suffering has to undergo training so that the correct āsanas can be performed in the correct way to cure the disease.

24

Yoga and āyurvedic medicine

Āyurveda is the traditional Indian science of medicine. 'Āyur' comes from the root 'āyuḥ', which means life, and 'veda' comes from the root 'vid', meaning to know, to understand. If you understand the body, the mind and the soul, this is known as āyurveda.

The origin of āyurveda is the *Atharva Veda* which, together with the *Ṛg Veda*, the *Sāma Veda* and the *Yajur Veda*, constitute the four Vedas – the sacred writings which are at the very root of Hindu thought and philosophy. Nobody knows when the Vedas came into existence. They are known as 'apauruṣeya': not given by man. Yoga too is apauruṣeya. Because these sciences are not man-made, they are universal and are meant for the whole of humanity. Brahmā was the founder of yoga, which is therefore as old as civilisation. Āyurveda is also as old as civilisation. It is the mother of all other systems of medicine, whether they be allopathic or homeopathic. In āyurveda you will find treatment of disease through remedies which give the same symptoms as the disease, as in homeopathy, and also remedies which give symptoms opposite to those of the disease, as in allopathy. Āyurveda uses both methods.

In the Vedas, we read: 'The fountain for all action is the perfection of the body.' And further: 'One who is a weakling cannot have experience of the soul.' Thus, the body is the fountain for the evolution of each individual. The aims of yoga and of āyurveda are almost the same. Both are concerned with self-realisation. The only difference is that yoga adopts a psycho-spiritual approach and āyurveda a physico-physiological approach. The cause of diseases, according to yoga, is the fluctuation of the mind, or chitta. For āyurveda, on the other hand, diseases are attributable to imbalances in the constituents of the body.

The five elements of which we are all made up are earth, water, air, fire and ether. The first element is earth, which is the ground for the production of energy. When the energy has been produced, its distribution requires space, which is the last element, ether. Earth and ether, the producer and the distributor of energy, are in themselves unchangeable and eternal; they change when they come into contact with the other three elements, which are air, fire and water. Āyurveda speaks of the three doṣas, or humours of the body, known as vāta, pitta and kapha, which are the air, fire and water principles as they manifest themselves in the body. Āyurveda explains that the imbalances in vāta, pitta and kapha disturb the equilibrium of the body and cause diseases to occur.

According to the philosophy of yoga, the disturbances take place on account of the imbalance of the three guṇas, or qualities of nature and mind in each individual's behavioural patterns. We met these three qualities in the story of Rāvaṇa, Kumbhakarṇa and Vibhīṣaṇa. They are sattva, rajas and tamas, or illumination, dynamism and inertia. These three qualities of nature disturb the mind, which in turn disturbs the functions of the body. The practice of āsanas and prāṇāyāma serves to create depth and to connect the innumerable parts of the body together.

There is no contradiction between the ways in which yoga and āyurveda explain the causes of afflictions. We have seven hundred muscles, three hundred joints, sixteen thousand kilometres of nerve current flowing in this human system, and about ninety-six thousand kilometres of blood veins, arteries, and capillaries. This human machine is so complicated, and it is very difficult to keep its many parts in good order. We don't know how many minor muscles are helping one major muscle to function – we don't even know their names. If the body is to move, there needs to be a current; this is the vāta current, the current of wind. Blood, too, has to circulate, and the current of blood is considered as pitta, the fire element. The blood is pumped to the various areas of the body, and in that flow, certain chemical energies are produced known as ojas, or lustre, in yoga, and tejas, or splendour, in āyurveda. This is nothing other than the element of fire, or electrical energy. Modern medical science also speaks of electrical energy running in our nervous system. Finally, kapha, the water principle, lubricates the body. Just as you need to send your automobiles for servicing, we need kapha in our system to service the body. Otherwise we would be like sticks – there would be no juice in our joints for movement at all.

The only difference between yoga and āyurveda is that in yoga tremendous will power is required. You have to generate your own energy to combat diseases. As many people lack the potency required to fight diseases, āyurveda gives tonics or vitamins to help the process. These tonics are medicines from the mineral, vegetable and animal kingdoms. The rasa, or taste, of certain tonics energises the body. Similarly, there should be rasātmaka-karma and rasātmaka-jñāna (action of taste, and knowledge of taste) in the practice of āsanas. The essence, or taste, of energy has to be felt in the fountain of your body when you are performing āsanas and prāṇāyāma.

It is said in both yoga and āyurveda that there are three types of disorder. Firstly, there are self-inflicted disorders. If we abuse our bodies, naturally we have to pay the price for it. These self-inflicted, self-invited diseases are known as adhyatmika-roga. Secondly, congenital diseases, known as adhidaivika-roga, are those that the children get on account of their parents. Thirdly, there is adhibhautika-roga, which means diseases caused by the imbalance of the five elements in our system. If your earth element is not in a state of balance, you suffer from constipation. If your water element is not balanced, you will suffer from disorders such as dropsy. If the fire element is not balanced, you will have gastric trouble with a burning sensation in the stomach. If you have a disturbed air element, you feel a bloated sensation in the abdomen, or rheumatism in the joints. If, all of a sudden, for no apparent cause, with no rhyme or reason, your body swells or shrinks, and then comes back to normal, this is due to imbalance of the ether element. The practice of āsanas helps to maintain the balance of the five elements and so to avoid the class of diseases known as adhibhautika-roga.

As in āyurveda, so also in yoga, there are vitamins. Patañjali says that the vitamins we need to maintain in yoga are faith, courage, boldness, absorption, and tremendous memory to understand exactly what is happening in us today, what happened yesterday, the day before yesterday and many days ago, with uninterrupted awareness. These are the five vitamins for the practitioner of yoga. If you haven't got these five vitamins, you are not doing yoga at all, but only bhoga. Bhoga is translated as satisfaction. You will remember that niyama begins with śaucha and santoṣa. Śaucha is cleanliness and santoṣa is contentment. Together they produce bhoga, which can be described as health of the body and harmony of the mind. But Patañjali does not finish with śaucha and santoṣa. He goes on to speak of tapas, svādhyāya and Īśvara-praṇidhana, which lead to liberation of the soul from the contact of the body.

Āyurveda starts from the body, and yoga starts from the consciousness. But from their different starting points, both serve to keep the body healthy, and both are mokṣa-śāstras, or sciences of liberation.

25

The practical approach

Modern medical science uses the drug cortisone which is considered to be the only drug which is applicable to all ailments. It could be said that the cortisone of yoga is the sight of the soul. Nevertheless, if you have a stomach problem, this is a practical problem which has to be dealt with practically. You have to work with a competent teacher to see why there is pain, what happens when you are doing which movements, what mistakes you are making in your postures, where the stress is when you are working, whether it is necessary to give stress to that point or whether it should be shifted elsewhere in order to nullify the strain. All these things have to be seen in your practice.

Suppose you have a boil on your leg, does the doctor immediately pinch the head of your abscess to bring out the pus, or does he first clean the surrounding parts of the body? If there is an internal cause creating the boil, there is no point just knocking the head off the boil, because all you are going to do is get another one. Similarly, in yoga, you cannot just knock on the point at which the ailment manifests itself. If you have a pain in your stomach, you should know that there are indirect processes connected with that ailment. You have to look at how the whole body is behaving. This requires only common sense to be understood. You have to strengthen the other parts of the body before you touch the injured part directly.

When you do āsanas, do not stretch that area directly, but first strengthen the other parts. You have to tell your teacher, 'I don't want direct pressure on that area.' Then nothing will go amiss. If there is a pain in a certain part of your body, you can't just think of quick effect. You have to train and tone the surrounding areas before you come to work on the affected area directly. Otherwise, you will aggravate the problem, and this will not be the fault of yoga. The cause of pain should be known and the yoga poses introduced judiciously in order to get rid of the pain. The indirect muscles have to be strengthened in order to work on the direct problem later. The teacher can observe from the outside and guide your work with his external eye, so that the surrounding parts are cleansed and strengthened before you come to work on your weak area from the inside.

In the majority of pupils, the intellect of the head is very strong, but the body does not react to the volition of the brain. Usually, their brain acts as a subject, but you have to learn to treat the brain as an object and the body as a subject. This is the first lesson yoga teaches. When that is learnt, the effect of yoga is very quick.

If you have a stomach problem, you can't dictate to it from the brain. There is no place here for the brain to act as a subject. If you use the brain, I become aggressive and say, 'Your stomach is suffering, not your brain!' I will be compassionate to your stomach but strong to humble your brain. I will say, 'Relax your brain! Let go!' This takes the tension out of the brain, and because of this lessening of tension, the stomach pain also lessens. Thus, psychologically we relax the brain and physiologically we work on the stomach. This makes the brain accept the pain, which becomes tolerable, and the energy that was wasted in tension is transformed into healing energy to work on the stomach. Then the injury can start to heal.

Perhaps it is more difficult for so-called intelligent people to treat the body as a subject, because they live in their heads. The yogī knows that he has a brain from the bottom of his foot to the top of his head. An intellectual person thinks that he is only in his head and nowhere else: his intelligence cannot spread beyond the brain to inhabit the rest of his body. But the yogī says, 'Diffuse that energy from the brain to the other parts of the body, so that the body and the brain may work in concord and the energy be evenly balanced between the two.' That is the beginning of the healing process, since the release of tension in the brain brings relaxation to the nerves.

I am often asked to give advice as to what exercises should be done by somebody suffering from this or that particular ailment.

I don't give advice. I only say, 'Work to get rid of the problems.' Advice has no value. I cannot recommend particular exercises. How would I know what type of effect it would have? That has to be seen in each particular case. Otherwise it would be like reading some books to know the effects of a medicine, then going to the pharmacy buying the medicine and taking it. One cannot read remedial methods in yoga books and treat pupils who come for relief on that basis. I cannot allow my pupils to do that. Books are only rough guides. If, as a teacher, you are confronted with particular medical problems, you have to seek advice from a senior teacher who has experience in handling such cases. Let them be your guides. Then you will be safe, and the pupils too will be in safe hands.

Consider the example of somebody with ankylosing spondylitis. If it is an old case and the bones are fused, it is difficult to make substantial progress. It is like a well-developed tree which cannot be pruned, whereas a sapling can be pruned according to the direction you want it to grow. If the disease is fresh, it can be acted upon like the sapling, but if the disease is very old, you have to be content to control it and see that it does not spread further. If it is fresh, act soon to tame it, and if it is spreading, act soon also to see that it does not spread further. Common sense has to be applied: alignment of the muscles with the bones, of the organs with the connecting fibres, of the inside, outside, back and front of the body, and the correct placement of the organs in their positions, all have to be observed while practising.

In your training, while doing trikoṇāsana, if you observe the line of the outer side of your body, many of you may find that the leg is doing half śavāsana: it is slanting from the foot to the hip. Look at yourselves in your own life, how each side of your body works. The knee and the thigh will be far away from the line joining the foot to the hip. That type of yoga is not going to cure diseases. The bone is the centre, and the muscles are the wings of that centre. The muscles should spread equally on both sides like the wings of a bird. If half the wing is cut, the bird is left with only one and a half wings and cannot fly. Similarly with one and a half muscles you cannot gain health in those parts and you cannot cure the disease. Each part of the muscle has to be divided equally so that the wings or the muscles are evenly spread on both sides. That is how to cure the disease.

If you are a teacher of yoga, you should have some background knowledge of the causes of diseases, how they develop and what parts of the body are affected. To be a yoga teacher is very difficult. Though you may know at once that such and such a person is suffering from certain ailments, if you do not know how to tackle it directly, you have to work from the periphery, by toning the muscles which are far away from the affected area. Make sure the muscles are toned all around – on top, at the bottom, at the side – then gradually come to work with the affected area. That way, risks are not involved. If the lumbar spine is affected, you have to train the cervical spine, the tail-bone, the sacro-iliac area and the thoracic spine. Only then can you come to the affected area. If you treat the lumbar spine directly in such cases, you not only take a risk, but also ruin your own name and spoil the noble values and benefits of the art of yoga.

A mature teacher of yoga attacks the spot directly if the disease is fresh, but if it is a long-standing problem, the teacher comes towards it from the other areas. First, make the other parts healthy, then come to the affected part to make that healthy in its turn. That is how yoga has to be taught in remedial cases.

These general ideas I have given, but I cannot give specific solutions for specific cases. One has to observe, learn under the guidance of an able teacher, then work with one's own individual discretion.

26

The art of prudence

Many yoga books describe the special cleansing techniques which are known as kriyās. But if you read the Haṭha Yoga Pradīpikā *carefully, you will find it is said that this is a therapy but not a part of yoga. The kriyās are given for diseases which are otherwise incurable, but many other means have to be used before these drastic measures are called upon – they are not for everyone. Modern medical science also has drastic measures. Cortisone is a drastic drug. If everything else fails, cortisone is given. Similarly, in olden days, when other methods failed, drastic treatment was given through the kriyās, but it was said that they should not be done by a healthy person.*

The same text says that the effects coming through these kriyās also come through āsanas and prāṇāyāma. Today, the majority of people are under the impression that haṭha-yoga means kriyās, but this is not so. Haṭha-yoga consists of āsana, prāṇāyāma, pratyāhāra, dhāraṇā, dhyāna and samādhi. The kriyās are something different, and are intended for people with abnormal diseases.

Some people clean the inner passages of the body using water, or a thread, or a cloth, according to the kriyās known as jala-netī or sūtra-netī or dhautī. But I do prāṇa-neti, or cleansing with the breath in prāṇāyāma. Why should I insert external things when nature itself has provided the thread of the breath? Therefore I say that sūtra-netī, jala-netī and dhautī are not necessary.

If a cloth is completely or partly swallowed and an abscess is formed in your stomach because the cloth was not completely clean, whom do you blame? How many people are able to master the technique for swallowing the cloth or for sitting in a bucket of water and drawing in water through the anal sphincter? Nature has provided the natural yoga system which is quite different from all this. That is why the ancient texts say these are drastic treatments, only to be given in drastic cases, and not for everybody. If you want to read this for yourself, you can look at Chapter 2, 21 of the *Haṭha Yoga Pradīpikā*.

If you take a sapling, you can observe how it grows. But if you pluck that sapling and put it in a different place each day, the plant dies. Similarly, you should not disturb your nervous system by these drastic measures. The kriyās are given for those who cannot be treated by other yogic means. If everyone does them, they may end up with other ailments at a later stage which are provoked by the misuse of their system.

The āsanas, too, should be used with due caution, taking into account the physical state of the practitioner. For example, when you move the arms up, it places a direct strain on the heart. So people with cardiac problems should avoid postures with the arms raised. The moment you lift the arms there is a strain on the heart, so we do not teach any standing poses for these pupils. This would be irritative and not helpful.

It is very difficult for me to explain to Westerners the difference between stimulative exercise and irritative exercise. Take jogging, for example. Medical science says that it stimulates the heart. But the difference should be made between irritation and stimulation. The heartbeat increases, but that does not mean that the heart is stimulated. Stimulating means energising or invigorating, but exercise can also be irritating or exhausting. In jogging, making the heart beat very fast is irritating to the heart.

In yoga we do back-bends, which are harder than jogging, but that does not irritate the heart because we don't get out of breath and our heartbeat is maintained in a rhythmic pattern throughout. So when we are teaching āsanas, we have to find out what is actually invigorating and what is not invigorating. After invigorating exercise there is absolutely no fatigue. Feeling nice after hard work means that the work was invigorating, but feeling exhaustion after ten or fifteen minutes is a sure sign that you are doing irritative exercise. This holds good in yoga too. For example, I might see one of my pupils teaching a pose such as ardha-chandrāsana in an irritative way, with tremendous strain, a tremendous load, a tremendous grip on the fibres. That is what I call the irritative way of doing yoga, so I may step in and teach the pose according to a stimulative approach.

Knowing very well that each pupil may have some physical defects or ailments, the teacher has to try to stimulate the affected areas and not to irritate them. Teaching yoga is very simple, but to teach yoga in the right way is very difficult. Though every pupil has the same structure of muscles, joints and tendons, that structure will be disturbed as a result of psycho-physiological imbalances arising through individual habits of use, and the teacher must take these disturbances into account. Therefore in large classes it is sometimes necessary to pick out the weaker persons and give them different exercises or special attention so that no injury can take place.

Returning to the example of pupils with a cardiac condition: the heart muscle is in a sac in the centre of the left side. When the sac turns outwards, that means that dilation of the heart has taken place, and cardiac diseases are certain. When we teach poses like setu-bandha-sarvāṅgāsana and viparīta-karaṇi, we move the sac to its original position. But when the arms are lifted, the heart is moved away from its normal position, so we advise pupils with cardiac problems not to do those poses where a strain is placed on the heart.

Nor do we teach them head-balance because the blood will rush very fast, and while going up into the pose they tend to hold their breath. The cardiac spine supports the muscles of the heart, so for cardiac patients the supporting muscles of the heart, which are situated at the back, have to be exercised and toned. Consider what happens after an earthquake. A heart attack is like an earthquake of the heart. What happens to the earth for several days after the initial shock? The tremors continue as, slowly, slowly, the earth finds its level. There is no second earthquake, but tremors continue while the earth settles back into its new place. The same thing happens after a heart attack. After the quake, the tremors continue while it finds its level. After the attack, the muscles which protect the heart are hard – the fibres of the protecting muscles are very tight. Because they have worked hard to protect the heart, tremors continue in the heart. Therefore, these protective muscles have to be made passive. We give poses which will make those muscles soft, and when they are soft, they can take a second attack without any problems because they are already relaxed. If you make the person do a head-balance, the muscles which are already over-tense will tense further in order to get the balance, and you can imagine what happens.

I have explained this in detail to give an example for your own good of how you have to approach the practice of āsanas in the case of physical ailments. Some people may take unnecessary risks. If others do it, let them take responsibility for what they do, but don't you do it. It is better just to relax the muscles and use bolsters for them to lie down and do śavāsana, with simple prāṇāyāma, and that is all.

Another word of caution, which applies to all women practitioners, is that it is always advisable to avoid the practice of inverted poses during the menstrual period. The natural flow at the menstrual period is discharge, and if the discharge does not take place properly, you have headaches and go to the doctor for treatment. If there is excessive discharge you also go for treatment. Now, if you do inverted poses at the time of menstruation, there will be a tendency to absorb instead of discharging. If the discharge is blocked by doing inverted poses, this may give certain coatings inside. To begin with, you may not find there is much effect, but as a result of the holding of the discharge through the effect of gravity, a coating may be formed inside, which may later lead to various diseases including cysts, cancer and so on. So it is advised not to do these poses at the time of menstruation. The poses which are advised at that time are forward bends, where the discharge is not at all disturbed. In these poses the natural flow is maintained and at the same time a physiological contraction takes place in the organ so that the drying is quicker.

On the other hand, when a man or a woman passes blood through the bowels, this is not a natural process like the physiological action of a woman's menstrual cycle. In this instance, the restriction concerning inverted poses does not apply. People suffering from piles do pass blood, but with the practice of inverted poses, this stops after some time. Blood does not accumulate because the pores of the skin are soothed, the affected areas are dried out, and healing takes place. Bowel motions are made easy, so there are no more ruptures and no more blood is passed. Thus, the human organism controls the blood flow in piles by closing itself up quickly. But in the menstrual period, it opens, and cannot be closed without leading to disease.

As an example, I shall give my own case. You may be shocked to hear this, but for nearly fifteen years, whenever I went to the toilet, I used to pass blood. This happened every time I went to the bathroom, and I could not get up from the toilet because of the irritation in my anus. So I went for a medical check-up, because I don't believe in operations unless I know for certain that they are necessary, and the tests showed that everything was perfectly healthy. Yet when I went to the bathroom, only blood came out, like tap-water. I never took any medicine, and it disappeared by itself after fifteen years.

I wonder how many people have the courage to face something like this. I have many top doctors among my pupils – people who are supposed to know about these things. They were scratching their heads, saying, 'We don't know why you are passing blood. There is no wound.' They told me I should have an operation and have the ring of the anus removed, so I said, 'If I don't know that there is a disease, tell me, why should I get it operated?' So they said I would just have to go on passing blood, and I said I would go on passing blood and wait to see when it would stop.

Another common complaint is psoriasis. Psoriasis is peeling of the skin. In the West, psoriasis may come to you because you wear a certain kind of socks, or clothes that have been in a drying machine. There are many possible causes. A healthy person can withstand them, but if there is some weakness in the blood, one may get infected. In my experience, though peeling takes place and rashes appear, which is very irritating, the cracks close soon if the person practises inverted poses both morning and evening, head-balance and neck-balance with variations, which may take about two hours. The quality of the blood improves and the cracks soon close. I do not claim that I can cure the disease, but as I have experienced this with many pupils I say it can be controlled and recovery is fast.

Now, concerning eczema, if it is a dry eczema then there is absolutely no problem, all the poses can be performed. When there is a wet eczema, you have to be very careful when you are working, to see that perspiration or the dripping of the affected area does not touch the other parts of the skin. But if I am asked whether yoga can be done or not, I say definitely it can be done; I have worked with both types of eczema.

I don't know if I still have the mark, but I was teaching an eczema patient long ago and the infection went into my body also. It was irritating for years. I also get lots of nail poison, because when I teach, the pupils grip my leg or other parts of my body, and their nails prick my skin. You know that Mr Iyengar sometimes hits his pupils to help them in their postures, but perhaps you do not know what I get from my pupils! I also get the pupils' imprints on my body. I had itching for two or three years. Nothing was visible, but the irritation was there, and I used to use an ointment of camphor and ghee which I would apply to stop the irritation. Then one day my wife had a bucket full of water. The end of the handle; where it curves round in a loop, had a sharp point. I didn't know the bucket was there, and I opened the door and walked straight into it. That sharp point hit exactly the part which was irritating, and a cupful of black blood came out and the irritation disappeared. It was so black in colour, and then the fresh blood started coming. I told my wife this had been irritating me all these years. These are the kinds of problems I have while teaching, though I do not normally speak of the diseases which come my way.

In America I have treated one case with AIDS, and the person decided to come to my Institute in Pune to undergo training, because he was not suffering from exhaustion any more. He said he could do all kinds of manual work which he could not do before practising yoga. My American pupils were thinking of opening a clinic for AIDS patients, to see what yoga can do, though I said to them not to go too fast. It is clear, then, that people suffering from eczema, psoriasis and similar disorders can all do yoga without fear, and without expecting any bad result.

Finally, I would like to give a counsel of prudence to teachers who want to apply for themselves practices they may have seen others using in a specific context. Suppose somebody comes to a class when I am teaching women in the sixth month of pregnancy, sees what I am doing and says, 'Oh, this is good yoga,' and goes away thinking they know how to work with pregnant women. They have not seen how I work from the third month to the ninth month. They do not know that I have a different way of working for each month, and then they go away and think that because they have seen me teaching certain poses to pregnant women, they know how to do it.

I have given this example of pregnancy, but many more could be given. For instance, I have been asked whether I recommend inverted poses for people suffering from glaucoma. I do have glaucoma patients perform these poses, but this does not mean it is something I can recommend. If I use these poses, it is because I know how to make a pupil do the pose. If a person suffering from glaucoma does a head-balance, the pressure increases. How the eyeballs should be, how the ears should be, how the breath should be, has to be learnt. If, like a doctor, I were to prescribe these poses for glaucoma, somebody else would immediately say, 'I want to serve humanity, so I am going to teach inverted poses to people with glaucoma.' This very thing happened a few years ago.

In Pune, I teach people with glaucoma and even displaced retina. I have taught a number of cases where the retina is not too severely displaced, so I am not nervous about it. If a patient comes to know that he is going to get a displaced retina, I can save him from getting the displacement. But having been bitten once I am very careful. A few years ago, while I was teaching head-balance to half a dozen people with glaucoma, a certain man joined my class and saw me working. He was not himself a glaucoma patient at all, but he saw me teaching and later he wrote me a letter, saying, 'Having seen you teaching head-balance to people suffering from glaucoma, I am also teaching it, and they are benefitting. Can you tell me what else I should teach?' I lost my temper. What can I do if such things go on? I am very wary about recommending exercises for physical conditions, because many people may say, 'I will also teach that.' But what is important is how it is taught. If you don't know how to do it, don't do it. This applies not only to the head-balance, but to many other āsanas which may put pressure on the eyes. Do not do it if you do not know. It is dangerous. In such a case, do forward bends only. That you can teach and no damage will be done; if the glaucoma remains the same, it will certainly not increase, so I am safe, you are safe, and those who do the poses will also be safe.

27

The healing art

The original idea of yoga is freedom and beatitude, and the by-products which come along the way, including physical health, are secondary for the practitioner. Nevertheless, we can observe how these by-products are brought into being and how the effects of the āsanas and prāṇāyāma percolate in the body, rejuvenating the cells and the cellular system. Because we can learn by observation how different physical and physiological effects are triggered by various movements, we can come to know that those are the paths which affect the other parts of the body.

This is traditional knowledge but the links in our tradition have been lost, and so have to be retraced by scientists and practitioners. The reason for the loss of the links is historical, and we should all know it. At one time yoga was practised by everyone, and at that time India was at peace – there were no invasions at all. But then, in the last thousand years, India has been the victim of land invasions from North, West and East, and finally also on its sea fronts. Its culture, its temples and places of learning went through periods of systematic destruction and undermining. Thus, many of our ancient traditions were lost and our links with them severed. Traditionally the knowledge was all there, but it has been lost and we have to work it out again. That is why we have to follow our own experience and find what I call the optimum possible movement which works.

Practitioners of yoga and research scientists have found many leads to connect us to the lost material. Having practised āsanas and prāṇāyāma for years, and having reached the optimum possible level in our practice, working with resistance, without resistance, observing and experimenting with our own reactions, it is possible for us to trace the meridians within the body and work on them on our own, without depending on another person's help to get treatment. Yoga is a subjective medical treatment which affects the various vital centres of the body.

It is a very complex subject. Take for example the notions of īda, piṅgalā and suṣumṇā which are the main channels of energy in our body. These can be related to the Chinese conceptions of yin and yang. Īda is yin (feminine), and piṅgalā is yang (masculine). These two channels of energy meet at certain places; they criss-cross in the system, and wherever they cross each other is a meridian point. When we practise the āsanas or prāṇāyāma, there is an interchange of energy between these two at the centres where they meet. These centres are storehouses of energy. When the optimum presentation of our body allows the correct uninterrupted flow of energy to take place through the channels of īda and piṅgalā, then at that time the hidden energy can be released from those centres to act for the healing of the various diseases from which the body is suffering.

When you have reached the optimum possibility of right movement and perfect action in each āsana, then consciousness will exist everywhere in your body whether you are aware of it or not. Yet it is only when intelligence is brought to bear that awareness is also awakened. When there are diseases you should know that that part of the body which is affected by the disease has lost its sensitivity. There are then various ways in which it can be rejuvenated through the practice of yoga. When we are doing the postures, energy is brought into those affected areas. Having understood this through our own experience in our own bodies, when correcting our pupils' poses we touch them at that point so that the energy may flow uninterruptedly into each area for the sake of a recovery.

My warning to you all is not to try to help where you know that you do not know anything. That is a risk. I have said several times, and again I have to warn you: teach only what you know. Do not teach what you do not know, taking others as guinea-pigs to make an experiment. Be a guinea-pig on your own self before you play with others. I tell you this because a yoga teacher is in a different position from a doctor when helping people. A qualified doctor gives medicine but does not come into contact emotionally with the patient. The doctor knows the symptoms, knows the causes of the disease and knows that certain drugs work for certain diseases. He or she prescribes the drugs and you go to a pharmacy, buy them and take them according to the prescription. If you improve, well and good. If you don't improve, the doctor tells you to go to a specialist and get examined. In healing through yoga, the teacher comes in contact with the pupil or patient, and from moment to moment sees their emotions and reactions. In yoga there is no intermediary like a pharmacy from whom to buy the remedies. You have to be very careful because you are playing with another life. The medical doctor is not so much playing with life as with medicine. If the drug does not work, the doctor says, 'Alright, I'll change the medicine.' But in yoga you cannot change the medicine; you have to go back always to the same principles. So you need to know how these principles are to be applied in any given case.

Some people say that I am a physical gymnast in yoga. It is unfortunate: only people who do not know the real depth of yoga can speak in that way. I have gone deep into my body; I am a subjective practitioner. I do not depend on acquired knowledge. I have the knowledge of experience. I know the depth of each āsana. I have to penetrate the duality between one muscle and another. Suppose I have a lower arm which is longer and an upper arm which is shorter. It may look very healthy, but it is deformed. The joint should be exactly in the middle and there should be no variation between the upper part of the body and the lower part. To reach this point is known as understanding. The āsanas help us to remove these dualities or dysfunctions in the body, mind and soul.

Take the example of someone suffering from buzzing in the ears. This is a practical problem of the patient, and needs a practical answer. It may be that there is some blockage of the ear. The bones may be too close together, or there may be pus in the ear. The person may be physically weak, or the wax of the ear may be unbalanced. The construction of the neck and the ear need to be looked at. I cannot know without seeing the person, but in general these problems can be helped by inverted poses such as sarvāṅgāsana, halāsana and setu-bandha-sarvāṅgāsana. These inverted poses do help, but if the pose is not taken correctly, instead of the sound being reduced, pain will also come. So the teacher has to be vigilant to see if pain comes in the ear while the pose is being performed. Ṣaṇmukhī-mudrā is also helpful, but to know how to insert the fingers into the ears is an art. It has to be tried, and by careful trial and error, one learns how to adjust the inner ears in the process. Tremendous skill and sensitivity in the fingers have to be cultivated to balance the inner ears.

I have a pupil in Pune who had this problem. She never used to answer the telephone because she could not hear. Her parents came crying to me some time ago saying, 'Our twenty-year-old daughter is deaf and we cannot marry her. Please do something to help her.' I said, 'What can I do? The child is deaf. But I shall try, and if I succeed, see that your girl gets married soon.' So I took the case and trusted that God would help me in my treatment.

Before I took the case the parents took her to an ear specialist who said, 'It must be operated on immediately because an eighty per cent closure has taken place. If it is delayed by a month or so it will be completely closed and there will be no chance at all after that.' The parents were my students, and I asked them why they had not told me before, when the problem started. They said they thought yoga might not be able to help, so they had kept quiet. Then I said, 'Alright, I have another pupil who is an ear, nose and throat specialist in Bombay. I will send your daughter to be examined by him so that he can give me the right picture.' He examined the ear and said, 'There is no doubt that an operation is necessary, but if Mr Iyengar is going to take her I can wait three months. If he can do something in three months, then we can stop the operation, but if he does not do anything in that time, do not delay, get it operated.'

So I handled the case. I started teaching her, and after three months he made tests again and there was a substantial improvement. This is something that medical science cannot believe. Even my daughter Geeta was surprised when I took on this case, saying, 'What are you going to teach, when it is that deep inside the ear?'

I have treated fungus of the ear and itching of the ear, and have cured these things. Naturally this was a little more difficult, but I took the challenge and started to work with her. For most of us, when we do head-balance or other inverted poses, the hole of the ear, which is normally circular, takes the shape of an egg – an oval shape. If it becomes oval, your head-balance is wrong. From this one example you can understand just how subtle you have to be in teaching. When I insert my finger in her ear while she is standing upright, performing tāḍāsana, I see how deep it goes. Then I watch similarly in head-balance, and the finger should go further than in tāḍāsana. If it does, then that head-balance is the correct head-balance which makes her completely serene and passive, so the block disappears and the hearing improves. I worked with her on other, more difficult poses, taking into account that she was very slim and very tall, so halāsana and sarvāṅgāsana would not help. The ears started opening, and the girl gave me the clue, saying that she felt it was opening. From that clue, I learned so much about many āsanas. After three months she went for a test and the doctor was surprised to find that the left ear was completely open and the blocked right ear had opened ten per cent more than before. So the parents said, 'Now the girl is better. Is it necessary to continue?' I said, 'Why not try another ten per cent? My responsibility is to help her to hear till she gets married, and after marriage she can listen to the voice of her husband. From then on, I'm not responsible!'

Then one day when I was teaching, the specialist from Bombay came to my class. During the class, I inserted my finger in his ear and told him, 'Your right ear does not hear properly.' He asked me, 'How did you know?' That is what I mean by art. You have to learn how to insert your finger. The ear is so delicate. I adjusted his ear and he said he could hear better. After the class he said, 'Mr Iyengar, yoga is not curing that girl. You are curing her!' Now the ear is forty per cent opened. She can hear the telephone. She can talk to anybody. So I told the parents, 'Marry her soon!'

How do you make the ear open? I can't explain. It is not so easy. You should know how to place the vagus nerves by doing shoulder-balance, and then after manipulating the vagus nerves you have to manipulate the nerves of the ears. Then it is possible to see a change. But in the case of somebody who is fat, and whose ear is small, for example, there is bound to be a buzzing in the ear because of the anatomical structure. Many things are involved. Such a person would have to come to Pune so I could see what I could do. I may fail also, but I don't mind taking a chance for the simple reason that if a second person comes I will start from where I stopped with the first person. Even though there may be no improvement with the first person, I will know how to work after that with other people. I will not be able to guarantee success for the first person but I can guarantee improvement for the others.

When I started teaching yoga I was a useless teacher. Circumstances or students demanded of me that I teach yoga, so I started teaching from the age of sixteen. When people started coming and asking me to teach, I used to get lots of headaches and diseases in my body. I took their pains and their sufferings into my own body. Then I used to do yoga with that pain in my body. I subjectively learned what those pains were. I subjectively learned the pains of others. And I subjectively experimented on my own body the effects of the āsanas and right and wrong movements, before giving these movements to them. This is how I became a good teacher.

You can only give what you yourself have experienced. If you wish to help others through the healing power of yoga, you have to put yourself at the service of the art and then through experience gain understanding. Do not imagine that you already understand and impose your imperfect understanding on those who come to you for help.

Remember that experience and the knowledge born of experience are a million times superior to accumulated and acquired knowledge. Experienced knowledge is subjective and it is factual, whereas acquired knowledge, being objective, may leave the stain of doubts. So learn, do, re-learn, experience, and you will be able to teach with confidence, courage and clarity.

Part Four

The Self & Its Journey

28

Return to the seed

We have described the eight limbs of yoga as the parts of a tree, proceeding from the roots to the flower and fruit. The spiritual development of the human being can also be likened to the growth of a tree from seed to full maturity. The quality of the growth of a tree cannot be seen in the seed, but it is hidden within it. The seed of the human being is the soul, within which the essence of our being is hidden. The soul in each individual is what causes that individual to grow, just as the seed causes the growth of the tree.

When the seed is sown, after one or two days it sprouts into a seedling. This seedling is known as dharmendriya. Indriya is an organ, and dharma is virtue, or essential nature. Dharmendriya, the organ of virtue, is the conscience. This sprouting or the seedling of the soul gives the first perception, a perception of virtuousness, an opening of the gate.

When the seed has thus opened, a stem grows out of it which is chitta, or consciousness. Then that single stem which comes out from the seed divides into various branches – one branch is the small self, known as asmitā; another is ego, or ahaṃkāra. Asmitā is awareness of individual existence. It is not yet ego. It is the awareness of the self, of 'I am'. Ahaṁkāra is ego – it is the sprouting of asmitā, the self, into action. As long as the self is not acting it is asmitā, but the moment it expresses itself in action it becomes ahaṁkāra.

As consciousness develops, it breaks into various branches. One branch is ahaṁkāra, or ego; another is buddhi, or intelligence; another is manas, or mind. As the tree continues to grow, further branches emerge which are the karmendriyas and jñānendriyas, the organs of action and senses of perception which come into contact with the external world and create thought-waves, fluctuations, deliberations, modulations, modifications. Like the leaves of a tree meeting the atmosphere, the individual self, the individual intelligence and the mind come into contact with the outside world and gather information which feeds back to the branches, the main stem or trunk of consciousness and the seed of the soul. Thus they act as a bridge to bring the inner body and the outer body in contact with each other.

This development from the seed to the stem to the branches and leaves is a natural process in each individual. If the leaves do not move at all, that means there is no exchange with the air, and the leaves wither up and the tree gets dry. The leaves are there to feed the whole tree. In the same way, our organs of perception and of action are meant for the cultivation of the inner body. Unfortunately, we usually forget the inner body and concern ourselves with the outer body only, because we only see the world outside and not what is going on inside the tree. We do not see how nourishment is drawn from the external atmosphere by the leaves and flows in the sap, protected by the bark, to feed the root and the whole tree.

Our organs of action and perception are there to gain knowledge and understanding and to culture the intelligence and the ego, thereby feeding the self and the original seed, the soul, which is the cause containing the essence of the whole. As the tree developed in an outward journey from the seed through the stem to the branches and leaves, the return journey must also be made from the leaves back to the seed. In practising āsanas, you feel the energy flowing in your system. You feel how it is working, how it is flowing. In the tree, the energy flows from the seed to the leaves, and as the leaves make contact with the air they feed energy back on a reverse journey through the branches and the stem to the root, and the root makes the tree grow further to produce the blossom, fruits and flowers.

The brain is at the top of the human body as the fruit is at the top of the tree. In yoga, we have to make the brain, the mind and consciousness become as objects. This is not to deny them – it is to culture them. European philosophy begins with the brain, the seat of thinking. Yoga begins with the seed. The brain, according to yoga, is the periphery of the consciousness. From there, you have to move inwards towards the root. Because we are too much in the head, we lose contact with the rest of our body.

Consciousness is always present in our finger, but most of the time we are not aware of it, so the consciousness of the finger is dormant. You should know the difference between consciousness and awareness. Consciousness exists everywhere in the body. When you are walking, if a thorn touches your foot, what happens? It pricks, and you immediately feel the pain, so you cannot say that consciousness was not there. But until the thorn pricked you, you were not aware of your foot. The consciousness in your foot was dormant, but the moment the foot was pricked, it was brought to the surface. To awaken that dormant consciousness is awareness. Your consciousness is six feet long, or five and a half feet long in your body – it is as long as your body is tall. But awareness is small. Awareness may extend two feet, one foot, one inch or half an inch. The yogī says that by practising āsanas, you can bring awareness to an extension equal to that of consciousness. This is total awareness. This is meditation.

When awareness fades, concentration fades, intelligence fades, and consciousness also fades. But the moment you are attentive, your intelligence is concentrated. This concentration is dhāraṇā, and when that intelligence and awareness do not fluctuate but remain constant, that is meditation. Because there is no interruption in observation, there is no interruption in the flow of intelligence, there is no fading of awareness, so the subject and the object become one. In dhāraṇā the subject and object are still separate – that is why you have to concentrate to bring back the subject to look into the object, or to draw the object towards the subject. But the moment the object dissolves into the subject and the subject forgets itself, this is samādhi. Then there is no difference between me and the object of my contemplation. The moment the object and the subject come together, there is no object, there is no subject; there is soul; there is the seed.

29

Patañjali's *Yoga Sūtras*

It is very hard for practitioners of yoga to know the depth of its meaning. We all know that stilling the mind is yoga. In olden days when the great sages and yogīs wrote their books, they gave the goal at the beginning of their teachings and then defined the methods of stilling the mind in order to reach that quietness. Some two thousand five hundred years ago, Patañjali wrote the Yoga Sūtras *which contain four chapters consisting of a hundred and ninety-six sūtras or aphorisms, in which a complete method is given whereby each individual can develop and be at one within himself.*

In the first two sūtras he says that when the mind is stilled, the self rests in its abode. If things were as simple as that, then Patañjali could have ended there. But he goes on to amplify those two sūtras with a hundred and ninety-four further sūtras in which he defines the technical ways of reaching that state. He begins by saying that when the mind is stilled, the self rests in its abode. But when the mind is not still, when the mind is wandering, when the mind is attracted towards external objects, the self follows the mind, and as it follows the mind, it cannot rest in its abode.

In the first chapter, Patañjali describes how the mindstuff gets attracted by things seen or heard, which create fluctuations or thought-waves in the mind. He gives various methods for stopping these fluctuations of the mind, adapted to differing individual capabilities and different levels of development, so that all practitioners can reach oneness between mind, body and soul.

The uncultured mind fluctuates because of habits of behaviour, so he gives methods of concentrating on the universal spirit of God, or on breath, or on those who have reached liberation through the practice of yoga, or on anything which is congenial to you. By following these yogic methods the practitioner develops a cultured mind, and in that cultured mind analyses correctly, reasons accurately, or without interfering with the objects of the external world, neither analyses nor reasons, but remains silent. When the cultured brain becomes quiet, there is a state of bliss, and in that bliss the practitioner experiences the core of the being.

More than two millennia ago, Patañjali realised the importance of the brain and described the front brain as the analytical brain, the back brain as the reasoning brain, the bottom brain as the seat of bliss (which, incidentally, corresponds to the findings of modern medical science, that the hypothalamus, situated at the base of the brain, is the centre for pleasure and pain), and the top brain as the creative brain or the seat of creative consciousness, the source of being, ego or pride, the seat of individuality.

Patañjali introduces ways of culturing the brain whereby its four parts are made passive; they are made to remain as objects like our hands and legs, so that they may become silent. When they are silent, there is absolutely no movement of the brain. Instead of being extraverted, the brain becomes introverted and begins to trace its source. This passivity has been experienced by all of us in moments of sleep where the brain does not function at all but remains as a thing. At that time one loses the awareness of oneself. Yogic philosophy describes this state as a spiritual plateau or spiritual desert, as when people come and go at a crossroads but do not know in which direction to go if there are no signposts. It is also a state of poise and peace.

Patañjali warns us not to be caught in this quietness. There is something beyond it, known as the seat of the very conscience. If you reach tranquillity of consciousness and get caught up in it, remember that there is a downfall known as yoga-bhraṣṭa, which means 'fallen from the grace of yoga'. This occurs when one gets caught up in this stage and imagines that it is the end of yoga. The practice of yoga must continue as it has to culminate, according to Patañjali, in the sight of the soul. So from fluctuation to stillness, stillness to silence, and silence to the sight of the soul is the journey of yoga. With intense effort and faith you have to recharge the battery of your intelligence to move through the vibration of the consciousness and find out where the vibration of consciousness ends. When you reach that state, you develop a mature consciousness known as seasoned or mature intelligence, which does not waver, and you become one with the core of your being. This is known as nirbīja-samādhi, or seedless samādhi.

This is the conclusion of Patañjali's first chapter, called *Samādhi Pada*, which is meant for people who have reached a certain level of spiritual development. It is clearly explained that this chapter is not for all, but for those who have reached the stage of development where they maintain an even attitude in all circumstances. It shows how these cultured souls can maintain that maturity in their being without interruption.

The second chapter is meant for those who have not begun their spiritual development, or who are just beginning. It speaks of the afflictions of the body which cause fluctuations in the mind. The pains of the body create fluctuations in the mind, so by countering the afflictions of the body one counters the fluctuations of the mind.

Now, as I have said, yoga is integration. The second chapter gives the background to understanding what integration is. We are made up of three tiers: the kāraṇa-śarīra or causal body, comprising the spiritual sheath; the sūkṣma-śarīra or subtle body, comprising the physiological, psychological and intellectual sheaths; and the sthūla-śarīra or gross body, comprising the anatomical sheath. The sūkṣma-śarīra or subtle body lies between the other two – it is the bridge connecting the body with the soul. When these two are connected, according to Patañjali, the dualities between body, mind and soul disappear.

At the beginning of the second chapter we read, 'Tapaḥ svādhyāya Īśvarapraṇidhānani kriyāyogaḥ': self-discipline, self-study and surrender to God together comprise the yoga of action (*Yoga Sūtras*, II, 1). When the body, the mind and the senses are cleansed by tapas (ardour and self-discipline based on burning desire), and when understanding of the self has been attained through svādhyāya (self-study), only then is the individual fit for Īśvara-praṇidhana (surrender to God). He has brought down his pride and developed humility, and that humble soul alone is fit for bhakti-mārga, the path of devotion.

Thus, Patañjali has neglected neither karma-mārga, the path of action, nor jñāna-mārga, the path of knowledge, nor bhakti-mārga, the path of devotion. He has given importance to all these three for the simple reason that each human being is made up of three parts: the arms and legs for action, the head for thinking, and the heart for devotion and surrender. Each individual has to follow these three paths. None is higher or lower than the others, and each requires its own particular kind of action.

This second chapter of the *Yoga Sūtras* is called *Sādhana Pada*, the chapter on practice, and Patañjali goes on to describe the various methods which can be used according to the level of one's development. These are the eight limbs of yoga, known as yama, niyama, āsana, prāṇāyāma, pratyāhāra, dhāraṇā, dhyāna and samādhi, which we studied one by one in Part Two of this book.

The third chapter is called *Vibhūti Pada*, the chapter on attainments. It speaks of the wealth of the effects of the practice of yoga, which may disturb the harmony of evolved souls because of the temptation of yogic powers. Patañjali describes the powers which may be gained from the practice of yoga. He gives about thirty-five effects which might be experienced, and which are an indication that one's practice is sound. If your practice is sound, he says, these are the effects you experience. If you don't experience any of these effects, that means your practice is imperfect. But these riches, these gifts that come through yoga, are also a trap. So he also teaches non-attachment.

Unfortunately, these results are sometimes described as supernatural powers, but they are not in fact supernatural powers at all. They are the sensitive achievements which come automatically through the practice of yoga. But the practitioner may get carried away by these successes, like someone who runs away from the wind and gets caught in a whirlwind. In order not to get caught in the whirlwind of what appear to be supernormal powers, Patañjali advises you simply to observe whether you have any of these qualities or not, and then to continue further the practice of yoga.

These powers and gifts are traps for the practitioner just as the joys and comforts of the material world are traps for an ordinary person. Patañjali explains that just as an ordinary person fights to get rid of afflictions, the yogī has to fight when he gets these powers, because they can become psychological afflictions. Though they may appear to be supernormal powers, they are not supernatural, but are simply the finest of the powers of nature. As the practitioner has developed sensitivity and intelligence, he experiences the effects of that sensitivity. These powers are normal, though they appear supernormal to people who have not developed that degree of sensitivity. But when you attain that sensitivity and these powers become normal for you, you have to be careful because that which you had not previously experienced becomes a temptation. It is like a celibate person who will be tempted by a woman. The newly experienced powers will be a trap for you and divert you from the true aim of yoga. This is why you have to develop non-attachment.

When pain and the fluctuations of the mind have been conquered, the practitioner acquires spiritual powers and gifts, which have to be conquered in their turn. Only when these are conquered is the spirit alone. When the soul is freed from the bondage of body, mind, power and pride of success, it reaches the state known as kaivalya, or aloneness, where the body and mind are as it were in quarantine and the soul is free. This is the subject of Patañjali's fourth chapter, called *Kaivalya Pada*, the chapter on absolute liberation.

30

Prāṇāyāma

Prāṇa means energy. Cosmic energy, individual energy, sexual energy, intellectual energy, all are prāṇa. It is even said that prāṇa causes sun and the rain to come. Prāṇa is universal. It permeates each individual as well as the universe at all levels. All that vibrates is prāṇa – heat, light, gravity, magnetism, vigour, power, vitality, electricity, life, breath, spirit, all are forms of prāṇa. Prāṇa is the hub of the wheel of life. All beings are born through it and live by it, and when they die, their individual breath dissolves into the cosmic breath. It is potent in all beings and is a prime mover of all activity.

Prāṇa and consciousness are in constant contact with each other. They are like twin brothers. It is said in yoga texts that as long as the breath is still, prāṇa is still, and hence the mind is still. All types of vibrations and fluctuations come to a standstill when prāṇa and consciousness are quiet, steady and silent.

Knowing this connection between breath and consciousness, the wise yogīs of India advocated the practice of prāṇāyāma, which is the very heart of yoga. The texts do not explain how prāṇa is released in our system, but the Purāṇas contain a marvellous story which I take to be an image of this process. I mentioned this story already in Part Two. Now I would like to look at it in more detail.

Thousands of years ago there was a war between the demons and the angels. The demons were very strong and were destroying the universe through their muscle power. So the angels became nervous, saying that there would be irreligion everywhere. They approached the creator, Brahmā, for help, but he said that he could do nothing for them, as he was the one who had given the demons their strength. He advised them to approach Lord Śiva. But Lord Śiva said, 'I also can do nothing. I blessed them and gave them long life.' So,Brahmā and Śiva went in their turn to Lord Viṣṇu for advice.

Now Lord Viṣṇu listened to them and considered the matter. He said to the angels, 'Go to the demons and say, "Let us churn the ocean, to draw from it the elixir of life, and let us share it to become immortal." Then, when this nectar of life comes out of the ocean, leave its distribution to me.' So the discussion took place between the demons and angels, and they agreed to churn the ocean.

To churn the ocean they needed a churning rod, so they brought Mount Meru to act as a rod. Then they needed a rope to move the mountain. Lord Viṣṇu said, 'Take my servant, Ādiśeṣa, the lord cobra.' Ādiśeṣa agreed to his master's words and said, 'You can use me as a rope to move the mountain.'

Into the ocean they dumped trees, creepers, grass and raw materials of the earth for churning, so that these materials would be mixed together and produce a new blend – the elixir of life. These raw materials represent the five elements of the body, namely earth, water, fire, air and ether. The demons, being strong, held Ādiśeṣa's head, while the angels held the tail, and they began to churn. The churning represents inhalation and exhalation in a human being. As they were churning, the mountain which they were using as a churning rod sank into the ocean because of its great weight, and they could not churn any more. As it was sinking, the angels prayed to Lord Viṣṇu, who appeared in his incarnation as a turtle (Kūrma) and crept underneath the mountain to lift it up so that they could churn once more. Viṣṇu incarnated as Kūrma in this story represents the seer or soul in each of us, which is a particle of the Universal Spirit. The seer or soul is known in Sanskrit as puruṣa. 'Pura' means a fortress, a castle, a town, a house, an abode, or a body. 'Īśa' means master or owner. Puruṣa, the soul, is lord of the body, which is its abode. The diaphragm, which is above the seat of the soul, is represented in the story by the base of the mountain, the mountain itself represents the chest, and the churning represents inhalation and exhalation. Lord Ādiśeṣa is a representation of suṣumṇā, the principal channel of energy in the body, and his head and tail represent īda and piṅgalā, of which we shall say more in the next chapter.

When the churning was taking place, the first thing to come out was a deadly poison, halāhala. Lord Śiva, full of compassion for humanity, drank it to save the human race from utter destruction, and his neck became completely blue. Then several jewels came out of the ocean, and lastly the nectar, jīvāmṛta, the elixir of life.

When the nectar came out, Lord Viṣṇu took the form of Mohinī, an attractive and beautiful woman, who danced and distributed it only to the angels. Thus, righteousness was established again in the universe. Similarly, when we breathe, we first get rid of the toxins of the body in exhalation, then inhale to draw in nectar from the atmospheric air.

In our body we have five elements. The element responsible for production of the elixir of life (prāṇa) is earth. The element of air is used as a churning rod, through inhalation and exhalation, and distribution is through the element of ether. Ether is space, and its quality is that it can contract or expand. When you inhale, the element of ether expands to take the breath in. In exhalation, the ether contracts to push out toxins.

Two elements remain: water and fire. If there is a fire, water is used to extinguish it. This gives us the idea that fire and water are opposing elements. With the help of the elements of earth, air and ether, a friction is created between water and fire, which not only generates energy but releases it, just as water moving turbines in a hydroelectric power station produces electricity. To generate electricity, the water has to flow at a certain speed. An inadequate flow will not produce electricity. Similarly, in our system, normal breathing does not produce that intense energy. This is why we are all suffering from stress and strain, causing poor circulation which affects our health and happiness. The current is not sufficient so we are merely existing, not living.

In the practice of prāṇāyāma, we make the breath very long. In this way, the elements of fire and water are brought together, and this contact of fire and water in the body, with the help of the element of air, releases a new energy, called by yogīs divine energy, or kuṇḍalinī śakti, and this is the energy of prāṇa.

Prāṇa is energy; āyāma is the storing and distribution of that energy. Āyāma has three aspects: vertical extension, horizontal extension, and circumferential extension. Through prāṇāyāma we learn to make the energy move horizontally, vertically and circumferentially to the frontiers of the body. Prāṇāyāma is the link between the physiological and the spiritual organism of man. As physical heat is the hub of our life, so prāṇāyāma is the hub of yoga. The *Praśna Upaniṣad* says that consciousness and prāṇa are twin brothers. Similarly, the *Haṭha Yoga Pradīpikā* says that where there is mind there is breath, and where there is breath there is mind. If you can control the breath, you can control the mind and vice versa, so you should learn to make the breath rhythmic through prāṇāyāma. But it is not to be practised without due caution, because it can make you or mar you. If your heartbeat is uneven, fear sets in and death may be near at hand. Similarly, if prāṇāyāma is unrhythmic, your energy is sapped instead of being enhanced.

Unfortunately, prāṇāyāma is often taught without the proper foundation. The *Haṭha Yoga Pradīpikā* says, 'When the yogī becomes perfected in āsana, when his body is controlled, then with the help of his guru he can learn to do prāṇāyāma.' When explaining the practice of yoga, though Patañjali speaks in general terms of the eight stages of yoga beginning with yama and ending with samādhi, he does not say, for example, that yama should be practised before pratyāhāra, or niyama before āsana. But when he begins the techniques of prāṇāyāma, he specifically says, 'Tasmin sati śvāsa praśvāsayoḥ gativichchhedaḥ prāṇāyāmaḥ': only after mastery of āsanas has been achieved, should prāṇāyāma, which is the art of regulating inhalation, exhalation and retention, be attempted (*Yoga Sūtras*, II, 49).

The next sūtra explains that inhalation, exhalation and retention have to be made precise. Patañjali says, 'Bāhya ābhyantara stambha vṛttih deśa kāla saṁkhyābhiḥ paridṛṣṭaḥ dīrgha sūkṣmaḥ' (*Yoga Sūtras*, II, 50). This is a very important sūtra, and it is worth looking at it in detail. 'Bāhya' means external, or out-breath. 'Abhyantara' means internal, or inbreath. 'Stambha' means control, and 'vṛtti' means movement. So the sūtra begins with control over the movement of outbreath and in-breath. Then we have 'kāla', which means time, 'deśa', which means place, 'sāṁkhya', which means number, and 'paridṛṣṭah.', which means regulated. The breath has to be regulated or made precise in time, space and number. Unfortunately, when you are taught to breathe on eight counts or sixteen counts, you can easily forget the last words of the sūtra which are 'dīrgha', long, and 'sūkṣma', subtle. We tend to concentrate on the length but forget the subtlety. The flow of breath when counting should not vary at all. Inhalation and exhalation should be long, soft, smooth and uninterrupted.

'Stambha vṛtti' is control of the movement. When there is no movement in the cells, the mind, or any of the vessels of the soul, that is known as kumbhaka. The *Haṭha Yoga Pradīpikā* speaks of antara-kumbhaka and bāhya-kumbhaka, or suspension of breath with lungs full and suspension of breath with lungs empty, as well as pūraka, inhalation, and rechaka, exhalation. It says we are to learn to channel the in-breath and out-breath without disturbing the body.

Patañjali also speaks of a fourth method in prāṇāyāma. The first method is inhalation; the second is exhalation; the third is inhalation-retention and exhalation-retention; and the fourth method is when effortful effort becomes effortless through conquest of āsana. At first, prāṇāyāma is deliberate and effortful, but only when it becomes effortless have we achieved mastery. This is kevala-kumbhaka, which means pure or simple kumbhaka – kumbhaka which takes place by itself and has become natural and effortless. In kevala-kumbhaka there is no thinking. There are no internal or external thoughts. In this spiritual prāṇāyāma, you cannot think of anything except aloneness.

Prāṇāyāma is at the frontier between the material and the spiritual world, and the diaphragm is the meeting point of the physiological and spiritual body. If, when you hold your breath, your mind sinks after some time, that is not kumbhaka. Even by counting 'One, two, three, four' you have lost divinity – you have lost peace. Remember that kumbhaka is not holding breath; it is holding energy. Kumbhaka is realising the very core of the being which is brought towards the body. You don't think externally and you don't think internally. Having controlled the movements which take place inside and outside, you see that in that silence, no thinking takes place. When you don't think at all, where is the mind? It dissolves in the self.

The *Haṭha Yoga Pradīpikā* says you consciously come to experience that state of oneness with the self through prāṇāyāma. When you are one within yourself, you become a king among men. It is an indivisible, absolute state of existence.

It doesn't require extraordinary intelligence to be honest, but to be dishonest, how cleverly we have to use our brain! Life has been made complex on account of our behaviour. But truth is simple, hence life can become simple. To bring back the complexity of mind to simplicity is the aim of yoga, and that simplicity comes by the practice of prāṇāyāma.

In the brain there is a tug-of-war between pure and impure consciousness. It is like the churning of the ocean. The same churning goes on between the intelligence of the inner or subconscious mind or heart, and the intelligence of the head or brain. A veil of darkness covers the consciousness of the head. If the brain gets clouded, you cannot see clearly. The practice of prāṇāyāma removes the clouds in the brain to illuminate us and bring clarity and freshness, so that we can see the right thing at the right time. Usually we see the right thing at the wrong time, or the wrong thing at the right time. But if the mind is wandering, make the exhalation soft and slow, and stay there for a while. Let your consciousness flow with your breath. Then the fluctuations will stop. You reach a single mind and the dual mind disappears. Then your mind is fit for meditation.

When you inhale, the self comes into contact with the body. Hence, inhalation is the evolution of the soul towards the body and the spiritual cosmic breath coming into contact with the individual breath.

Exhalation, from the point of view of physical health, is the removal of toxins from the system. From the psychological point of view, it quietens the mind. From the spiritual point of view, it is the individual breath in the person coming into contact with external cosmic breath so that they are one.

Exhalation is the surrender of our ego. It is not the expulsion of air but the expulsion of ego in the form of air. In exhalation, you become humble, whereas pride comes in inhalation. Prāṇāyāma is also spiritually dangerous if you do not know how to practise it. To say 'I can hold the breath for one minute!' is pride. To learn prāṇāyāma is to learn and to understand the movement from attachment to non-attachment, non-attachment to attachment.

31

Energy and divine grace

We have spoken of prāṇa. Now let us look at īda, piṅgalā and suṣumṇā. These are the three principal nāḍīs, or channels of energy in our body. Physiologically, they have one meaning; psychologically they have another meaning.

Physiologically, piṅgalā corresponds to the sympathetic nervous system, īda to the parasympathetic nervous system, and suṣumnā to the central nervous system. The sun is the producer of energy, and piṅgalā is known to yogīs as the sūrya-nāḍī, the nāḍī of the sun. It begins from the solar plexus. Īda is the chandra-nāḍī, the nāḍī of the moon, and has its origin in the brain. The coolness which is attributed to īda in the *Haṭha Yoga Pradīpikā* is explained by modern medical science as being linked with the hypothalamus, which is at the base of the brain and is the centre responsible for keeping the body temperature even. So the hypothalamus is the lunar plexus, from which īda descends, as piṅgalā ascends from its seat in the solar plexus.

There is a tremendous connection between the sympathetic nervous system and the parasympathetic nervous system. Medical science says that if the sympathetic nerves are acting, the parasympathetic nerves are at rest, and if the sympathetic nerves are affected, then the parasympathetic nerves supply energy so that the balance of the body mechanism is maintained. Likewise, the yogīs say that īda and piṅgalā work together. One is heat; one is cold. One is like the sun and carries solar energy; one is like the moon and carries lunar energy. If the sun were there for twenty-four hours a day, what would be the fate of the the world? What would be the fate of humanity? We would all die! The moon, giving only the reflected energy of the sun, has a cooling effect. That is why there is day and night. Similarly in our body, when piṅgalā is very active, īda says 'The heat is increasing, so let me act.' This corresponds to the action of the sympathetic and parasympathetic nervous systems.

The coming together of īda and piṅgalā in our system, like the fusion of fire and water, produces a new energy. This is the energy of suṣumṇā, which is known by the name of kuṇḍalinī. Suṣumṇā corresponds to the central nervous system, and this divine energy, produced by the fusion of īda and piṅgalā, is seen physiologically as electrical energy.

The sympathetic and parasympathetic nervous systems are semi-controllable or semi-voluntary, like the respiratory system. Normal breathing is automatic, but you can also control it. Similarly, through the various movements of the āsanas, you can increase the energy of the sympathetic nervous system, or you can increase the energy of the parasympathetic nervous system. The amount of energy in the central nervous system cannot be controlled in this way. You cannot say, 'Let me increase my electrical energy.' But the fusion of the two energies of īda and piṅgalā produces energy which is stored in the body and can be released to supply electrical energy to the central nervous system. Through the central nervous system, this energy can be supplied to every part of the body.

Suṣumṇā exists everywhere, not just in the spine, because the central nervous system exists everywhere. Suppose you are stretching the index finger in an āsana; if the outer edge of the index finger stretches more, and the inner edge does not stretch so much, that means the solar energy is flowing more and the lunar energy less. You must pay attention to the lunar energy so that the excess of solar energy is nullified. When, by the practice of āsanas, the solar and lunar energies are balanced and made to run evenly in the system, they are nullified, and the practitioner feels a new sensation and a new energy flowing between the two. This is the energy of suṣumṇā, which runs through the whole body.

This is the interpretation of īda, piṅgalā and suṣumṇā on a physiological level. Now let us look at them psychologically. Consider the nature of clay. The earth powder is the primary cause out of which various forms or designs are made. It may be a jar; it may be a vase; it may be a bowl. All these things can be formed from the powder of the earth. If you want to change the form, you have to break the one you have and return to the original powder before you can make a new design. Now, chittavṛtti-nirodha, restraining the movements of the mind, according to Patañjali, is not yoga; it is just the beginning of yoga. 'Chittavṛtti' means the movements of consciousness – the various forms consciousness can take, like the clay taking various shapes. Primary gold can take various shapes such as bangles, necklaces, earrings, nose-rings, bracelets, anklets, and so on. But in order to change the anklet into a bracelet, it has to go back to the primary gold, just as the clay has to go back to the powder before it can be modelled into a new form. Similarly, if you want to understand what the self is, you have to understand the nature of consciousness, not the nature of the movements of consciousness.

'Vṛtti' means movement. 'Nirodha' means restraint and 'chitta' means consciousness. So 'chittavṛtti-nirodha' means restraint of the movements of consciousness, but not restraint of consciousness itself. Until you stop the movement, how can you understand the nature of the powder or the primary gold and how the powder brings the various forms? You have to go to the cause. As the powder is the cause for the forms of the clay, and as the primary gold is the cause for the various objects which it can produce, so chitta, consciousness, is the cause for chittavṛtti, the movements of consciousness.

Through restraint of the movements of consciousness, a space is created between thoughtlessness and thoughtfulness, between emptiness and fullness. Observe that. By observing the space between the two, you realise that chittavṛtti is different from chitta – the movements of consciousness are different from consciousness itself. Patañjali says that when consciousness becomes quiet, when that contemplative state of attention has come, through āsana, prāṇāyāma, dhāraṇā and dhyāna, then the consciousness realises that it has no light of its own, because it cannot act and witness at the same time. It is dependent on the reflection of the light of the soul. That is the subtlety of the character of consciousness.

In the first chapter of the *Yoga Sūtras*, Patañjali speaks of the fluctuations of consciousness, but not of the essential characteristic of consciousness – what consciousness really is. He only explains in the fourth chapter the essential characteristic, or dharma, of consciousness, and that dharma is that, like the moon, it has no light of its own. Consciousness realises that it has no light of its own and that it is dependent on something else. It realises that it is borrowing its light from the core of the being. Chitta, the mind, draws its light from ātma, the soul, just as the moon borrows its light from the sun.

When consciousness, which has acted as a subject up to now, realises that it has no light of its own, but has borrowed the light from the soul, then it surrenders to the soul. The fluctuations of consciousness cease. Restraint has now naturally taken place. Then the brain remains quiet. It becomes empty. It ceases to behave as a subject and becomes an object, passive, receptive. The moment the brain is transformed into an object, there is a diffusion of our intelligence equally everywhere. That means that īda and piṅgalā, the sun and the moon, are balanced and give way to the third light, which is the divine force of suṣumṇā known as kuṇḍalinī.

The *Haṭha Yoga Pradīpikā* says that kuṇḍalinī only awakens when grace falls on you, so all effort is useless unless that grace comes. What does Patañjali say about this? He says you do not know at what time grace will fall on you, so you must prepare everything so that you can accept grace when it comes. He says, 'Be physically firm, mentally stable, and spiritually ready to receive it.'

Patañjali has explained very well that the vehicles of nature – the organs of action, the organs of perception, the mind, the intelligence, the consciousness – are all there to serve their lord, the soul. If you know how to use them, then they become your servants. These vehicles are there as friends to help the self, but if the self does not know how to use them, they become the masters of the self, and that is the cause of unhappiness, affliction, fluctuations, disturbances. Patañjali speaks of 'bhoga' and 'apavarga'. 'Bhoga' means 'caught in the web of the world'; 'apavarga' means 'caught in the force of the divinity'.

Āsanas and prāṇāyāma are the fountain to create and maintain that divine energy of kuṇḍalinī, which is equal to cosmic energy.

If the inner energy of your mind and the energy outside are one, then no harm will come to you. You are a divine individual, and will accept that light without any damage. But it can happen that when the divine power comes to you through yoga, because of some weaknesses in your inner energy, it may bring unhappiness, or disturb the balance of your body. So you should prepare yourself so that when the divine light comes to you, your body, your mind and your nerves are able to receive it. We have spoken of the healing process in yoga, but remember that yoga is a preventive as well as a curative system. And we are speaking here not only of the body, but of mind and the soul also.

At school, the teacher gives the lesson and all the pupils hear the same words. But though they all hear the same words, and maybe even write the same words in their notebooks, they do not all get the same marks. One gets a distinction; one gets a second class pass; one gets third class; another fails. They all hear the same words, and all make efforts, but they grasp or understand the lesson differently, and nobody knows who is going to get a distinction. The power of kuṇḍalinī is like the mark. Some may just get pass marks. Even if you don't do yoga, sometimes the divine light comes, like a pass mark. But if you work a little more, you earn more, and if you work still more intensively, you will earn more still. This energy has to be earned, and when it comes to complete maturity, it is like a tree which gives fruit. The essence of the entire tree is in the fruit. Similarly, the essence of your entire practice is contained in this divine energy known as kuṇḍalinī.

In a yoga class, you may get this energy because the teacher touches you and you receive something of the teacher's vibration. This is like pass marks. But is it temporary or permanent? If it is only temporary, you have to work to make it permanent. Then the divine force remains eternally in you.

If the health of the body, of the mind, of the nerves and of the intelligence are completely ripe, then that light remains eternally. Until then, it will come and go. Some trees give fruit, some give no fruit. Some give tasty fruit, some give sour fruit, and it may be that on the same tree one fruit will be very tasty and others not. That divine kuṇḍalinī is the fruit of the tree. It depends on your own practice and on divine grace. So work to attain it, and if it comes, hold on to it. No divine force can awaken without divine grace. You may have the will to get it, but if there is no grace, it will not come. That is why I said you must hold on to it. If the grace has come, continue your practice, and don't allow it to disappear.

32

Meditation and yoga

Meditation is not something that can be expressed in words. It must be directly experienced in one's life. Nor can meditation be taught. If someone says he is teaching meditation, you can immediately know that he is not a yogī at all.

Meditation is to bring the complex consciousness to simplicity and innocence without pride and arrogance. No spiritual experience is possible without ethical discipline. Ethical and spiritual practices go together, to drink the nectar of divinity. Hence, the ethical disciplines of yama and niyama are essential if one is to follow a spiritual path.

We have already seen that yoga is divided into three parts. Yama and niyama are one part. Āsana, prāṇāyāma and pratyāhāra are the second part. Dhāraṇā, dhyāna and samādhi are the third part. Yama and niyama are the discipline of the organs of action and the organs of perception. They are common to the whole world. They are not specifically Indian, nor are they connected to yoga alone. They are something basic which has to be maintained. In order to fly, a bird needs two wings. Similarly, to climb the ladder of spiritual wisdom, the ethical and mental disciplines are essential.

Then, from that basic starting point, evolution has to take place. In order for the individual to evolve, the science of yoga provides the three methods of āsana, prāṇāyāma and pratyāhāra. These three methods are the second stage of yoga, and involve effort.

The third stage comprises dhāraṇā, dhyāna and samādhi, which can be simply translated as concentration, meditation and union with the Universal Self. These three are the effects of the practice of āsana, prāṇa and pratyāhāra, but in themselves do not involve practice. Because there are tremendous variations in practice, there are going to be variations in the effect. If you work for two hours, you get only two hours' salary. If you work for eight hours, you get eight hours' salary. If you show initiative, you may get a rise in salary. That is how business works. Dhāraṇā, dhyāna and samādhi are like that also. If you work diligently on āsana, prāṇāyāma and pratyāhāra, you will receive your reward of dhāraṇā, dhyāna and samādhi, which are the effects of that practice. They cannot be practised directly. If we say that we are practising them, this means that we do not know the earlier aspects of yoga. It is only by practising the earlier aspects that we can hope to arrive at their effects.

What does Patañjali say about the effect of āsana? 'Tataḥ dvandva anabhighātah': the dualities between body and mind disappear (*Yoga Sūtras*, II, 48). What does he say about the effect of prāṇāyāma? 'Tataḥ kṣīyate prakāśa āvaraṇam. Dharaṇasu cha yogyatā manasaḥ': the veil covering the light of knowledge is removed and the mind is made a fit instrument for concentration (*Yoga Sūtras* II, 52 and 53). And what of the effect of pratyāhāra? 'Svaviṣaya asamprayoge chittasya svarūpānukāraḥ iva indriyāṇāṁ pratyāhāraḥ': through pratyāhāra the senses stop importuning the mind for their gratification and are withdrawn from their external pastures in order to help the mind on its inner quest (*Yoga Sūtras*, II, 54). Thus, these three practices lead the practitioner to dhāraṇā, dhyāna and samādhi. Patañjali has coined a special word for dhāraṇā, dhyāna and samādhi. It is saṁyama, or total integration.

Dhāraṇā means attention or concentration. It is a way of focusing attention on a particular chosen path, region, spot or place within or outside the body. Dhāraṇā is control of the fluctuations of consciousness to focus it towards a single point. In dhāraṇā one learns gradually to decrease the fluctuations of the mind so that one ultimately eliminates all waves or tides of consciousness and the knower and the known become one. When consciousness maintains this attention without altering or wavering in the intensity of awareness, then dhāraṇā becomes dhyāna or meditation.

When oil is poured from one vessel into another, it maintains a constant, steady and even flow. Likewise, the flow of attention and awareness should remain stable and constant. This steady awareness is dhyāna. Dhyāna is the way of discovering the greater self. It is the art of self-study, observation, reflection and sight of the infinite hidden within. It begins with the observation of physical process, then involves watchfulness of the mental state, then blends the intelligence of the head with that of the heart to delve deep in profound contemplation. By this profound contemplation, the consciousness merges with the object of meditation. This conjunction of subject and object makes the complex consciousness simple and spiritually illuminated. The effect of yoga is that you are kindled with the light of knowledge and keep yourself completely pure with an innocent mind, not with an arrogant mind. That is the beauty of the wisdom of yoga: it is wisdom with innocence, not with arrogance. This is the effect of meditation: arrogance, pride and ego are transformed and transfigured towards humility and innocence, which lead towards samādhi.

To spread the soul equally from the heart of its abode towards its frontier is the meaning of samādhi. Samādhi is not trance. If a person goes into a swoon, is that samādhi? If it were, samādhi would have no meaning at all. The definition of samādhi is to remain conscious and experience the state of sleep. What does this mean? In sleep, you are not aware of anything. Only when you get up, you say, 'I had a sound sleep.' That in you which said that you had a sound sleep is the seer, the soul. The practitioner of yoga tries to keep the mind, intelligence, consciousness, organs of action and organs of perception a hundred percent passive, consciously. We have three levels of consciousness: the subconscious, the conscious and the unconscious. The yogī brings all these three facets of consciousness into a single state of consciousness known as super-consciousness. Where there is no subconscious and no unconscious, but only consciousness, this is samādhi. We cannot easily attain this because we have not even penetrated these three levels of consciousness, so we have to go slowly and start from the visible things to approach the invisible before we jump to the things which we do not even know or understand.

I have said that yoga means to bring together, to join, to unite.

This means bringing together what God has given you – the body, the mind and the soul. There is a tremendous disintegration in each individual between body, mind and soul, and the art of yoga was given by the sages of antiquity to bring together these disturbed vehicles of the self, so that humanity as a whole might develop oneness between them.

How is it that in India, where we have six hundred million people, very few are attracted by meditation? And how is it that by contrast so many Westerners are attracted by meditation? My colleagues in yoga work with you in a certain way because you cannot control your nerves. You are always under stress. To work is a stress. To sleep is a stress. To go to the toilet is a stress for people in the West! You are almost always under stress, so you are given what may be called passive meditation, and when you are made to remain silent for a while, you think you have reached yoga, or that your kuṇḍalinī has awakened! Easterners are more relaxed, so to tell them to do this kind of meditation has no meaning. On the contrary, they have to be taught to be more active, and that becomes an active meditation for the East.

It has become almost commonplace to hear people say that they are practising meditation. And they think they can practise meditation in isolation from the disciplines of yoga which come before, which are yama, niyama, āsana, prāṇāyāma and pratyāhāra. Remember that the river which runs from the mountain to the sea flows as a single unit, and that it will then evaporate, form into clouds and come back as rain to fill the river again. Similarly, the river of the body, the river of the brain and the river of the mind are all one, flowing from the soul to the skin and back to the soul. Do you say that you are only interested in one part of the river and not interested in another part? Just as the streams which begin from their source come together and flow into one great river connecting them all and joining the mountain to the sea, so also the entire human system forms a single river which runs from the soul to the skin and from the skin to the soul.

How can you say that you are interested in the river of the mind or the river of the soul while neglecting the river of the body? How can you discard some of the limbs of yoga, saying that they are merely physical, while meditation is spiritual? Meditation is not separate from yoga, nor is āsana separate from yoga. If you accept one part of yoga, which is meditation, how can you discard the other parts, such as āsana, prāṇāyāma, yama, or niyama. If you discard the other steps, why do you not discard meditation also?

Your body has several limbs. Which part do you neglect, and which part do you take care of to maintain it in good health? Each and every part of our body, of our mind, of our brain, is equally important. It is the same in yoga. You cannot separate the various limbs or aspects of yoga, saying, 'This one is important; that one is unimportant.' Each and every part of yoga is equally important, though many people mistakenly say that meditation is the highest.

By looking at the tree, one can know the health of the root or the disease of the root. You and I, who are not at all evolved like the great sages of antiquity, cannot penetrate the root, the seed, the core of the being, but have to look at the periphery (the body and its functions, the brain and its functions, mind and its functions) so that from these outer layers we can go deep to know the root of our very being and discover whether that root is healthy or not.

The art of yoga begins with a code of behaviour in order to build up moral conduct, physical conduct, mental conduct and spiritual conduct. Without knowing the letters of the alphabet it is impossible to learn to read or write. Similarly, without knowing the alphabet of yoga, which is yama, niyama, āsana, prāṇāyāma, pratyāhāra, dhāraṇā, and dhyāna, it is impossible to live in the abode of the self. Hence my request to you all is to understand the depth of yoga by starting from the periphery, so that you can reach the seed. It is only a few very extraordinary and exceptional people who are able to begin from the very core of the being.

33

The nature of meditation

Meditation is integration – to make the disintegrated parts of man become one again. When you say that your body is different from your mind, and your mind is different from your soul, that means you are disintegrating yourselves. How can meditation bring you back to integration if it is something which separates the body from the brain, the brain from the mind, or the mind from the soul?

If closing the eyes and remaining silent is meditation, then all of us are meditating every day eight or ten hours in our sleep. Why do we not call that meditation? It is silence, is it not? In sleep, the mind is stilled, yet we do not say that sleep is meditation. Do not be carried away – meditation is not so easy; it is like a university course. At the races, many horses run, but only one wins the cup. So also, we are all running in meditation but the winning post is far, far away from us because we have not conquered our senses, our mind, and our intelligence.

There are three transformations which take place in meditation. At the very beginning of his *Yoga Sūtras*, Patañjali says that stillness of the mind is yoga. Later, he says that when a person is trying to still the mind, there is an opposition which occurs as new thoughts or new ideas arise in the mind. There is a tug-of-war between restraint and the rising thoughts as they come together. When there is restraint of thought, after a little while some new thoughts are born in the gap. How many of us have caught that gap between the restrained thought and the rising thought? The space between the restrained thought and the rising thought is a moment of passivity. In that moment there is a state of tranquillity, and a person who can increase that pause, that space between the restrained thought and the rising thought, is transformed towards the state of experience known as samādhi.

Restraint of thought in itself is not samādhi, as you may think. When you can increase that space between the restrained thought and the rising thought, a third experience comes to you, known as ekāgratā-pariṇāma. Probably you have not heard that Patañjali speaks of nirodha-pariṇāma, samādhi-pariṇāma and ekāgratā-pariṇāma in meditation, describing the transformation from a state of restraint to a state of tranquillity, and from that state of tranquillity to a single uninterrupted point of awareness (*Yoga Sūtras*, III, 9, 10, 11 and 12).

'Pariṇāma' means change, or transformation, and 'nirodha' means restraint. You may have read that 'ekāgratā' means concentration. 'Ekāgratā' is a compound word with two parts. The surface, or colloquial meaning of 'ekāgratā' is concentration. When the wandering mind is brought to a state of restraint, this is ekāgratā, or dhāraṇā. 'Dhāraṇā' means to hold, but to hold what? It means concentration, but concentration on what? Patañjali says that when you learn to realise the space between the restrained thought and the rising thought, by prolonging that space you reach 'ekāgra'. 'Eka' means one, 'āgra' means base. So what is ekāgra? It is the core of the being, the soul.

Ekāgratā-pariṇāma is the state where the mind, the body and the energy are completely focused towards the one base which is known as the core of the being. Everything is drawn towards the soul like iron filings drawn towards a magnet. When you have realised this prolonging of the tranquil state where the rising thoughts and the restrained thoughts come to an end, at the culmination of the process of stilling the rising and restrained thoughts, the consciousness and intelligence are drawn as if by a magnet towards the core of the being. To live in totality with your energy, your intelligence and your consciousness as one single unit, knotted to the core of the being, is meditation. How many of us are so sensitive as to reach that level? Are we really sensitive?

Through the practice of yoga we gain awareness. If you cannot maintain that level of awareness in your everyday life, that means there is a barrier in you. How can awareness change? How can it fail? If there is no cloud between us and the sun, then the sun is full and we can see it very clearly. Only when a cloud comes in the way can we not see the sun. So what is meant by awareness? It is the light of intelligence shining. How can it change unless something comes in the way? How can it diminish unless some thoughts set in?

Meditation is like the weather. Yesterday the sun was not shining. Today the sun has come. What was happening yesterday? The weather was cloudy. Does that mean the sun was not there? Of course it was there, but the clouds came between it and us. And today, the clouds have gone. Meditation is like that. 'Tataḥ kṣīyate prakāśa āvaraṇam': the veil covering the light of knowledge is removed (*Yoga Sūtras*, II, 52). 'Āvaraṇam' means covered, so the light was covered by thoughts. A thought covered the soul as a cloud covers the sun so its rays cannot penetrate. The soul could not meditate; the sun's full rays could not reach the earth. Today the rays reach the earth because the clouds are not there. In the same way we have to find out what mechanisms come into our meditation, how our mind behaves, how the consciousness reacts, how the intelligence reacts, what thoughts come between us and the pure light of the soul, what thoughts come between us and awareness, inside and outside. When we become aware inside and outside, we can have the experience that meditation and physical action are not separate, that there is no division between body, mind and soul.

You may practise meditation and develop awareness when you are sitting quietly in a park, and it comes quite easily. But when you are busy working, your life gets dominated by thought and it is hard to have total awareness. When you practise āsana, prāṇāyāma and pratyāhāra, you learn to be totally aware – you develop awareness in your whole body while you are engaged in action. Then you can become totally aware in all circumstances. In a park, while you look at a tree, you forget yourself and you are one with the universe. Why can't you learn to be one with the universe of your own world – that is to say, your self and your body? This way of looking at daily life is total awareness, total integration and total meditation.

A person who meditates is free from time. Probably many of

you do not know what time is. We all know the word 'moment'. The moment does not move. The moment is stable, but our mind does not see the moment – it only sees the movement created by the succession of moments. We see the succession of moments like the spokes of a wheel. The moment is the hub of the wheel and the movement of moments is the spokes. In meditation, the person who has mature intelligence lives in the moment and will not be caught in the movement of moments.

The movement of moments is seen in the waking thoughts, the rising thoughts and restrained thoughts. The person of mature intellect tries to live in the moment without being caught in the movement of rising and fading thoughts. The movement is the past and the future; the moment is the present. The practitioner cultures his mind, his intelligence and his consciousness to live in the moment, and as each moment moves on to the next, he goes with the moment but not with the movement. That is meditation.

Have you ever looked at railway tracks? The wheels of the train run on two parallel rails. Consider these rails, one as a thoughtful flow, the other as a thoughtless flow. In the human machine we also have a thoughtless and a thoughtful flow, and our mind is rolling on these two rails. The yogī knows how to keep the rails parallel and to remain thoughtfully thoughtless, not thoughtlessly thoughtful. As long as he remains thoughtfully thoughtless, no second thought comes into his mind. The moment he becomes merely thoughtless, it is as if the welded joints, or the fish-plates which keep the rail joined along its length, come apart. Then there will be an accident. Similarly, if the thoughtful state and the thoughtless state are running equal and parallel, then there is a single thought, and you are living in the moment. If there is a slight change and a nut is removed from your attention or from your awareness, then an accident takes place. An accident is a mental disturbance, a mental block, so you have to maintain yourself in the state where no nuts are removed from the rail of thoughtful thoughtlessness.

Patañjali says God is He who is free from afflictions, who is not affected by actions, who is ever fresh and new. His actions have no reactions, and He is free from pains and pleasures. A liberated person is one who has undergone afflictions in life, and has conquered them. Such a person cannot become a God, or what you might call a God-man or a Bhagwan. We cannot become Gods, though we can become divine. And that divinity of life where the pleasures of the world and the pleasures of the spirit are evenly balanced is only possible to a man whose intellect is equal to the light of his soul. He alone can know the meaning of meditation. He is a meditative man. You and I are runners in meditation, but have not reached the goal.

34

From body to soul

At the culmination of yoga, there is freedom from the bondage of the body. Many people think that they can attain this by meditation alone, in a way which is unconnected with the body. But only the doer can find out whether the feeling in meditation is of isolation, or of absolute aloneness, or of fullness. I say you have to proceed through the practice of āsana and prāṇāyāma, and this is why some people call me a physical gymnast in yoga, as if I did not keep insisting that the aim of yoga is the sight of the soul! Through the performance of āsanas, I become totally involved and find oneness of body, mind and soul. For me this is active meditation.

Although āsana is sometimes described as physical gymnastics, this is a quite mistaken description, because āsana means pose, and after posing, reflecting and reposing. Āsana is not just exercise. You have to observe that the fibres of the skin are exactly parallel to the fibres of the flesh, so that action and cognition are brought together and the mind can feel there is yoga, or contact. Yoga means union, or connection. If the mind, through the perceptive organ of the skin, does not feel you are present in the āsana, then it is merely physical.

To understand this more clearly, we can consider the four stages of practice in yoga which are described in the ancient texts. The *Haṭha Yoga Pradīpikā*; the *Śiva Saṁhitā* (another important haṭha-yoga text) and Patañjali himself all speak of four types of practitioner in yoga.

In a beginner, the mind will always run on the surface, which is the physical body. At this stage you have to work with dhāraṇā, or concentration. Your mind is completely dismembered; you don't know what to do. So we teach awareness of the various parts of the body: first look at the foot, then come to the ankle, connect the ankle with the foot, then look at the knee, connect the knee with the ankle, connect the knee with the foot, then come to the hip, connect the hip with the knee, the ankle and the foot, then come to the lower torso, the upper torso, the armpits, the neck, the face, and so on. In this way, through the teaching of āsanas, we bring the vastness and multiplicity of the intelligence from a state of divided concentration into a single concentration. But still we are working on the surface level of the physical body.

The second stage is to make the mind feel the action. First we simply asked the pupil to concentrate on the different parts of the body in relation to one another. Now we say, 'Feel the mind while you are doing it. Is the mind moving with you, or is the mind not moving but only observing, watching?' At this second stage, we say, 'There, go with your mind! Let your finger also go with your mind. Let your knee also act with your mind.' There is a difference between bringing the mind to the different parts of the body as they move, and asking the mind to move with the body. The first stage is called ārambhāvasthā, the state of beginning. The second is ghaṭāvasthā, the state of the body. First you did not know the body; you only knew the ankle, the knee, and so on. Now you must know the body as a whole, through the mind.

When the mind has known the body, then comes the third stage, known as parichayāvasthā, acquaintance, or the state of intimate knowledge. Here you bring the intelligence to acquaint itself with the body. As two people are introduced to each other by a third person, so the mind introduces the body to the intelligence, which is the third vehicle of the human being. The mind says to intelligence, 'Look at what is happening here. Let me introduce you to my knee. Let me introduce you to my ankle. Let me introduce you to my arms.' That is parichayāvasthā, acquaintance – acquainting the intelligence, through the mind, with the body. It is like the person who introduces you to me. After introducing us, this third person disappears and you and I become friends. So the mind disappears and the intelligence and the body become one.

Then when acquaintance has come, through the intelligence,

we arrive at the fourth stage – niṣpattyavasthā, the state of perfection or ripeness. When the intelligence feels the oneness between the flesh and the skin, it introduces the self, the ātman, saying, 'See what I have done! Come and see!' Because you are then perfect in the pose, see that as you introduce the body, the mind, the intelligence and the self, they all run parallel together in the presentation of the āsana. This is freedom from the body. The body is forgotten in that moment because everything is flowing at the same speed and in the same direction. Patañjali says in the third chapter that the yogī's body should move as fast as the speed of his soul.

But if you forget the body before you go through the earlier stages, you will never reach that point. That is the problem. Until the finite is known, how can we touch the infinite?

Part Five

Yoga in the World

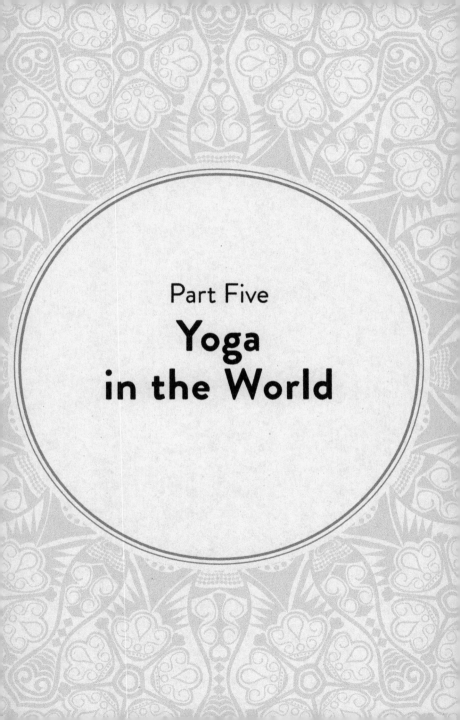

35

Yoga as an art

Yoga is known by almost everyone as a philosophy or as a path, but very few know that yoga is also an art. No artist can define his own art: what art is can only be expressed through art itself, and not by words.

The sages of ancient times distinguished between knowledge of the world and knowledge of the soul. Knowing that man exists as a physical, mental and spiritual being, and realising the importance of these three levels, they developed various arts to work on the trinity of man rhythmically, systematically and uniformly.

The six basic arts of Indian tradition are yoga, wrestling, archery, drama (including dance), music and economics. Arts can be of many kinds, including useful arts, healing arts, fine arts, performing arts and so on. The art of yoga embraces all these levels and is thus the fundamental art. Through yoga, the human being comes into contact with the soul; thus yoga is a spiritual art. Each āsana has an exact geometrical and architectural shape; thus it is also a fine art. Yoga brings health and happiness to the practitioner; thus it is both a healing and a useful art. When the beauty and harmony of the āsanas are appreciated by onlookers, yoga also becomes a performing art.

Three qualities are required if one is to become an artist. One must have aptitute, or the ability to acquire mastery of the art; one must have tremendous love for one's art in order to work on it with determination, effort and concentration, and one must have imagination and creativity to develop the art along new and unknown paths. What is known today was unknown yesterday. Every day there is new knowledge, but the unknown remains vast because the universal is vast. The unknown is the area which artists must explore in order to refine their art. While living in a normal social environment, artists must at the same time show new vibrancy and bring about hitherto untapped transformations in order for their art to live.

Lord Śiva is the founder of yoga, which he first taught to his wife, the goddess Pārvatī. He is also Naṭarāja, the lord of the dance. Yogīs and dancers alike pay respect to him, for he gave humanity this twofold knowledge so that human beings might experience the holy spirit of divinity in each and every cell of their bodies and find uniformity in diversity, impersonality in personality.

There is a beautiful story of how Lord Śiva invited Lord Viṣṇu to see his dance of destruction and creation which is called tāṇḍavanṛtya. Lord Viṣṇu was seated on Ādiśeṣa, the lord cobra. As Lord Viṣṇu was observing the movement of Lord Śiva, his body became heavy, and Ādiśeṣa was gasping for air. When the dance came to an end, his body became light. Ādiśeṣa asked Lord Viṣṇu what had made him become so heavy, and what had made him become so light. Lord Viṣṇu replied, 'I was totally absorbed in the dance of Lord Śiva and my body started vibrating, which caused heaviness. As soon as the dance was over, I came back to consciousness and became light.' Ādiśeṣa, realising the keen interest of his master in the art of dance, said, 'Sir, if the dance pleased you so much, why should I not learn dance and please you also?' And Lord Viṣṇu said to him, 'A time will come when Lord Śiva will ask you to write the *Mahābhāṣya*, the great commentary on grammar. At that time you can learn dance.' Now the author of the *Mahābhāṣya* is none other than Patañjali, who also studied dance as well as writing a treatise on medicine and the *Yoga Sūtras*. He is considered to be an incarnation of Ādiśeṣa.

The yogī believes in nivṛtti-mārga, the inward path of renunciation; the dancer believes in pravṛtti-mārga, the outward path of creation. Yoga is jñāna-mārga, a path of knowledge; dance is bhakti-mārga, a path of love. The difference between yoga and dance is that yoga is a perfect art in action, whereas dance is a perfect art in motion. In dance there is external expression through movement, whereas in yoga, though there is an intense inner dynamism, to the observer it may appear static. The movement may be very slight, but the action is tremendous.

We are all caught up in the web of lust, anger, greed, infatuation, pride and jealousy. These are emotional upheavals that come to us in our day-to-day lives. The dancer uses these emotions and transforms them into artistic expression. The yogī works to conquer them as recommended by Patañjali: 'Maitrī karuṇā muditā upekṣāṇām sukha duḥkha puṇya apuṇya viṣayāṇām bhāvanātaḥ chittaprasādanam' – to cultivate friendliness, compassion, joy, and indifference towards happiness and sorrow, virtue and vice, is conducive to mental peace (*Yoga Sūtras*, I, 33).

The yogī and the artist alike need to respect the body. Without shape and form, without grace and without strength, one can neither be a yogī nor a dancer. If you are an artist, remember that whatever themes you are presenting in your artistic expression, they all depend on the internal experiences and actions with which a yogī also works. If as an artist you also practise yoga – if you are also in touch with the internal levels of your being – you will develop a vast range of expression and your art will become what is known as 'satyam, śivam, sundaram', true, auspicious and beautiful. Art then becomes divine and is known as yoga-kalā, the art of auspiciousness. Art without this inner depth is known as bhoga-kalā, or art for pleasure. Art for pleasure has its value, of course, but if the intensity and devotion disappear, it can easily degenerate into kāma-kalā, or art for sensual gratification.

What is needed is a blend of bhoga-kalā and yoga-kalā. If there is only bhoga-kalā, the art is merely sensual and not uplifting, while if there is only yoga-kalā, it is too elevated and austere to be of value for society. To move, educate and inspire people, these two levels of art need to be combined and blended together so that all may live in the perfect light which illuminates the consciousness. Then there is a vivid vibrancy which enables each of us to live in the field of the soul, so that this mortal body may drink the nectar of the immortal soul and the art may become divine.

36

On teachers and teaching

It is relatively easy to be a teacher of an academic subject, but to be a teacher in art is very difficult, and to be a yoga teacher is the hardest of all, because yoga teachers have to be their own critics and correct their own practice. The art of yoga is entirely subjective and practical. Yoga teachers have to know the entire functioning of the body; they have to know the behaviour of the people who come to them and how to react and be ready to help, to protect and safeguard their pupils.

The requisites of a teacher are many, but I would like to give a few words for you all to catch, understand and work on. Later you can discover many more. The teacher should be clear, clever, confident, challenging, caring, cautious, constructive, courageous, comprehending, creative, completely devoted and dedicated to knowing the subject, considerate, conscientious, critical, committed, cheerful, chaste and calm. Teachers must be strong and positive in their approach. They must be affirmative to create confidence in the pupils, and negative within themselves so that they can reflect critically on their own practice and attitudes. Teachers must always be learning. They will learn from their pupils and must have the humility to tell them that they are still learning their art.

The relationship between teacher and pupil is like that between husband and wife, and like that between father and son. It is a very full and complex relationship. As in the relationship between husband and wife, which is one of closeness, teachers must ardently strive to see that their pupils do not fall, and to help them throughout their practice. At the same time, as between a father and a grown-up son, though there is relationship there is also distance. The job of the teacher is to protect and guide the pupils so that they may not fall from the path they have to tread. And the pupils' job is to see that what they have been given is maintained so that they do not slip into their own pitfalls. There is a two-way avenue between pupil and teacher involving love, admiration, devotion and dedication.

I remember very well that when India was under the power of England and France, Indians who had visited Europe used to put a notice in their houses proclaiming 'France returned' or 'England returned' as if they were extraordinary and privileged persons. The same thing is happening now in yoga. Students from the West come to India and 'India returned' yogīs are teaching yoga all over the place. It is indeed unfortunate that people take courses for a short while, then proclaim themselves to be yoga teachers. God alone knows how much experience they have or what is the quality of their work. People who go to them are also responsible because they do not put pressure on the teacher to find out whether the teacher has knowledge or not. Pupils also should have eagle eyes to watch their teachers.

Today, many people call themselves gurus, yogīs or yoginīs. This is wrong. Teachers should not be called gurus, and gurus are not to be seen merely as teachers. A guru is one who removes darkness and gives light. One who protects his or her pupils always so that they may not become victims of circumstances, and makes them work more and more so that they develop humility, is a guru. The role of the guru is to act as a bridge. Having experienced the truth, the guru is there as a bridge to help others towards God. The guru is an instrument of God, whose power moves in him or her, to shake those who do not yet understand the spiritual value of life, and to bring them nearer to God.

To live spiritually is to live in the present moment. When you are practising, as long as no other thoughts come to you, for that much time you are spiritual. The moment your mind wanders elsewhere, maybe to a person you have seen on the street, or to something somebody said to you in the office, then even if you are practising yoga at that moment, it is what is going on in your mind that is important, not what you are doing.

Yoga gives firmness of body, clarity of intelligence, cleanness of heart. That is peace, and by looking at that peace, others will learn. Cultivate that supreme strength of peace, joy and delight. Then others, seeing the joy in you, will say, 'I want to enjoy too.' You are a true helper of society when the pupil comes to you, instead of you going to him. Then it is a pure teaching and a pure message.

In my method of teaching, because I take you through a lot of poses, I keep you for two or three hours, or sometimes four hours, without allowing your mind to go elsewhere. Those who have worked with me have all experienced this. When I take a class for three and a half or four hours, do the pupils know that four hours have passed? No. So I have kept them in a spiritual state for four hours. If, out of twenty-four hours, they remain spiritual for four hours, I can say I have done some good in this world!

Suppose I were to ask you to do a meditation, to close your eyes and remain in silence, and suppose I also were to close my eyes. Could I know what was going on in your mind? Perhaps you would call that spiritual, but I would say there is no spirituality there because your mind will be wandering elsewhere. That is not my method of teaching. I teach externally, but in doing so I am keeping your internal organs in a state of single-pointed awareness for four hours at a stretch. So I don't need a certificate to say whether this is physical yoga or spiritual yoga. When I am teaching I know that for four hours your mind has not been allowed to wander. And when I teach I make you full – fully aware of your body, your mind, your senses and your intelligence.

I am very active in the classes I give. Does that mean I am not meditating? You may meditate sitting in a corner, but I am moving everywhere and I am meditating. What is the difference between the two? Sitting in a corner and closing the eyes is not necessarily meditation – it may be just emptiness. Some people say I am a physical man because I touch my pupils' bodies to correct them when I am teaching and ask them to stretch here or to stretch there. Yet at the same time I am aware inside and I am aware outside. As you sit with your eyes closed, you are aware inside but you are not aware outside. I too see within, but I also see outside with the same light. Otherwise, how could I correct so many people when I am teaching? If they make mistakes, I go immediately to correct them. So I am integrated when I am teaching fifty people or three hundred people. When one becomes completely integrated, that is meditation. How can I not be meditating when I know three hundred people's mistakes?

But when you close your eyes and say you are meditating, you don't even know your own mistakes. I could simply sit there saying, 'Do it this way. Do it that way,' but that would be creating a polarity between my pupils and myself. Instead, if the pupils are going wrong, I go and correct them, because they also should see the light that I have seen.

Now I don't mind finding fault with my own pupils who are teaching. Sometimes I give classes with fifty or sixty people. Thirty to thirty-five of them may be teachers and the rest students. When I look at them for a few minutes, I can see that they are teaching without practice. I am talking about my own pupils now, so you should appreciate what I am saying. When that happens, the first thing I do is to give them what you might call shock treatment. When the teachers say that they are not practising but nevertheless know what they are doing, I tell them that they should stop teaching if they do not practise for themselves. In the West, people go to classes without ever testing the calibre of the teacher. As the master tests the pupils, so too the pupils should test the teachers' standards before accepting them as teachers. A medical man cannot give medicine without undergoing proper training. So the pupils must give medicine to their teachers if they know that their standards are not up to the right level. This is known as an ethical discipline. Teaching with practice is ethical, but it is unethical when teachers teach without clarity in their postures.

Yoga cannot be learnt through lectures. Yoga has to be taught by precept, and in teaching, practical things are involved. It is very easy for pupils to find out whether the teacher is good or not. I cannot blame the teachers, but I blame the people who go to them without judging the standard. The moment the pupils start judging, the teachers will come to know that they are observed. This will make them realise how little they know and they will practise more and probably become good teachers. So I leave it to the students to decide.

There is very little value in teachers' certificates. The value is in the teacher's way of approaching teaching. The world is pure; ātman is pure, but unfortunately the people living in the world are very corrupt. As yoga became more popular in the West, many people started teaching yoga, claiming to teach the Iyengar method. Some used my name, and unfortunately still use it, to teach things which I myself never taught. When yoga came to be taught officially in England under the auspices of the Education Authorities, many people applied to be accepted as teachers, claiming that they had been trained by me, when this was not so. When the Authorities discovered that some of these teachers' methods were different from mine, they wanted assurance that teachers employed by them were indeed trained by me or by my senior pupils. This is why I introduced certificates for teachers, so that a uniform system could be maintained and so that no confusion might arise through one method of teaching being mixed with another. Through the certificates, at least you know who are my genuine students who have trained directly under me. Beyond this, the certificate has no special value. If teachers want to go further in their education in their chosen field, they can go on to get advanced certificates, as in other fields of education. But if you are happy with your primary education, be content with it. If you want to continue with secondary education, be content with that also. If you want to go on to do a PhD or even more, then that is up to you, but the important thing is not the certificate. What is important is whether you are sincere, whether you are humble, whether you are compassionate. You have to be compassionate as well as merciless. The two have to go together, but you must know where to be compassionate and where not to be compassionate in order to help the pupils with their problems.

If you are a teacher, do not go beyond the frontier of your knowledge. If pupils are overstretching, or if you do not know, then tell them you are the one who is teaching, and they should follow you. In this way, you can lead your pupils at a speed which you are sure of. Then you will get confidence. Yoga is a soothing thing. Even if I know the soothing action of a pose when I perform it, I also know the excruciating action it may have for you. In naṭarājāsana, for example, I know how to relax even in the stretch, but my students don't know how to. They experience fatigue. They do not allow the energy to flow. They block the energies in order to get the pose, and then they call it overstretch. I call it understretch. You all overstretch the brain and understretch the body. The tension and fatigue in that instance are in the brain. People tire first in the brain. The body takes longer. You should know which kind of fatigue it is.

The pupils who work so hard and so desperately in a pose that they become hard and tense are doing the āsana compartmentally. They do not know how to stretch evenly everywhere. If you overstretch on one side, that means you are dehydrating that part. You may be a beginner teacher, and you may have advanced pupils, but this need not be a problem. Who is to measure the overstretch? Overstretch means excruciating pain. The fatigue in the overstretched part comes immediately; it does not come afterwards. If there is no pain when you think you are overstretching, then it is only a mental block. You think, 'I am overstretching; I should not overstretch,' and it is that very thought which prevents you from going further in the presentation of the āsana.

When my body is tired, I say my body is tired; I never say that I am tired. If my brain is tired, I do halāsana and get back the energy, and if my body is tired, I do half halāsana and rejuvenate the cells. Maybe when you are tired, you do standing poses. You are already tired and then you overstretch in the standing poses, so naturally you get even more tired. You should use your discrimination – what to do, how much to do, and when to do it.

Now I shall ask you a question. When should a teacher end the class? If you are a teacher, when should you tell your students 'That is enough for today'? Everybody knows how to begin, but nobody knows how to end the class. It is important to know exactly when to end. If the pupils can't take more than I have asked, I say to them, 'Stop!' This is how I bring the class to an end. You may think a person has got tremendous energy, but you should know when he cannot proceed further. Do you look at the pupils' skin when they came into the class, to see what colour it is, and then again when they leave the class, what the colour is, and in between, what the colours are and what changes and transformations take place? As a teacher, do you observe all these things? I can say by looking at the skin that this person or that person cannot take it. The art of teaching is also to know when to stop. If you know when you have to make the pupil stop, then I can say you are a mature teacher. It is not a question of what you are giving. Perhaps you are giving a great deal because you want to build up a personality cult, or because you are afraid to stop.

And without innovation you cannot become an excellent teacher. Some bodies may have a long neck. Some may have a short neck. Some bodies may have a very narrow chest at the top and broad at the bottom. Others may be broad-chested at the top and narrow at the bottom. The spine may be very strong, or the spine may be very weak. And I have seen people who are tremendously intelligent, but with no connection to their body.

By coming into contact with people and knowing their emotional disturbances, I learn the poses which give emotional stability. I learn what exercises and what type of āsanas work on the liver, what works on the spleen, what works on the kidney, what works on the heart. I work on my own to discover how to stretch the liver, how to contract it, how to give lateral movement to the liver or to the stomach or to the intestine. This is how I have learned, and this is how I continue to learn. So I also have to be a creator at the time of teaching.

There are two types of teaching. One is explaining according to your intelligence. The other is knowing the weakness of your pupils, and how you have to explain in order for them to understand your meaning. That demands creativity. I have developed both kinds of teaching: I can give from my brain, and I can also receive the weakness of their brains and bodies and introduce a new style in order to make them understand and do well. That is the secret of my teaching.

When I was young – when society did not respect me at all – I was a pessimist. People called me a madman. But now, over fifty years of trials and errors have brought me to the point where I have clarity in what I am doing and in what I am teaching. Human failures there will be. Even greatly evolved people have made mistakes. I have taught many spiritual people in this world: scientists, artists, philosophers, saints, scholars. Do you think I do not learn from them? I am still a learner.

The first thing for a teacher to remember is that all the pupils who stand in his presence are as important as himself. Those who have trained under me become my children. Now my problem is how my children are going to look after my grandchildren!

Glossary

Most of the terms in this glossary are Sanskrit words, names of persons, deities, or legendary figures, or titles of scriptures or other ancient texts. Words in **bold type** in the definitions are words which have separate entries in their own right to which it might be helpful to refer. Entries in *italics* are either anglicised forms or Hindi words.

The 'ch' form has been used in preference to the 'c' form in words such as chakra (cakra), brahmacharya (brahmacarya), chitta (citta) and so on, in order to correspond more closely to English pronunciation. For ease of reading, compound words such as bhaktimārga and indriyasaṁyama have been hyphenated to give bhakti-mārga, indriya-saṁyama, and so on. For the same reason, compound words which are the titles of literary or sacred texts have been separated out. Thus we have *Bhagavad Gītā* and not *Bhagavadgītā*, *Atharva Veda* and not *Atharvaveda*, and so on.

abhiniveśa — clinging to life and fear that one may be cut off from all by death

abhyantara — internal; in-breath

abhyāsa — constant and determined study or practice

āchārya — master, teacher; one who propounds a particular doctrine

adhibhautika-roga — disease caused by the imbalance of the five elements, earth, air, water, fire and ether within the human system; injuries caused by living beings or creatures such as snakes, tigers and so on

adhidaivika-roga — disease transmitted genetically from parents to children, or due to past deeds (fate); disease caused by planetary influences

adhyatmika-roga — self-inflicted physical or mental disease; disease caused by misuse of the human system

adhyāya — study

Ādiśeṣa — the primeval serpent, said to have a thousand heads and represented as forming the couch for **Viṣṇu** or as supporting the entire world

ahaṁkāra — the ego; literally the 'I-Maker'; that part of our being which is active and self-conscious

ahiṁsā — non-violence, not merely in the restrictive sense of refraining from killing and from violence, but in the positive and comprehensive sense of love embracing all creation

amṛta — nectar

amṛtamanthana — nectar-churning, the subject of a story in the **Purāṇas**

ānanda — bliss, joy

ānandamaya-kośa — the spiritual sheath of joy, the core of the being – the innermost of the five sheaths enveloping the soul

see also **kośa, śarīra**

añjali — the hands joined in prayer

annamaya	composed of food (anna); material
annamaya-kośa	the anatomical sheath of nourishment; the gross material body – the outermost of the five sheaths enveloping the soul *see also* **kośa, śarīra**
antara	interior, inside, internal
antara-kumbhaka	suspension of breath after full inhalation
aparigraha	freedom from hoarding or collecting, absence of greed and of possessions beyond one's needs
apauruṣeya	revealed; not given by man
apavarga	emancipation
ārambhāvasthā	state of commencement, beginning, undertaking; the first stage of the practice of **yoga**
ardha	half
ardha-chandrāsana	half-moon pose – a pose in which the body and one leg are extended horizontally while standing on the other leg with one hand touching the floor and the whole body in one vertical plane
artha	means, utility, use, advantage, cause, motive; wealth as one of the objects of human pursuit
āsana	posture – the third stage of **yoga**
asmitā	'I'-principle; sense of individuality, awareness of pure being

āśrama	stage of life; there are four **āśramas**, each with its corresponding field of activity *see also* **brahmacharya, gārhasthya, sannyāsa, vānaprastha**
asteya	abstinence from stealing
Atharva Veda	one of the four **Vedas** or sacred Hindu scriptures, consisting of magical chants
ātma, ātman	soul, innermost Self, life principle
ātma-dhyāna	meditation on the greater Self
ātma-saṁyama	integration of the soul
ātman	*see* **ātma**
Aurobindo, Śrī	Indian nationalist and religious leader (1872–1950)
avasthā	state *see also* **ārambhāvasthā, ghaṭāvasthā, niṣpattyavasthā, parichayāvasthā**
avidyā	ignorance
āyāma	a movement involving length, expansion, extension, restraint, control, stopping
āyuḥ	life
āyurveda	knowledge of life; hence: the science of health, medicine
bāhya	external; out-breath
bāhya-kumbhaka	suspension of breath after full exhalation

bandha	lock, bondage, fetter; binding, contraction; a posture where certain organs or parts of the body are contracted and controlled
Bhagavad Gītā	the Song Divine, the sacred dialogues between **Kṛṣṇa** and the warrior king Arjuna – one of the source books of Hindu philosophy, containing the essence of the **Upaniṣads**
Bhagwan	blessed; the blessed one
bhakti	worship, adoration
bhakti-mārga	the path of devotion and surrender to the Supreme God
bhakti-yoga	the way towards realisation and union of the individual with the Supreme Soul through adoration, and devotion to the divinity
bhauma	of the earth; terrestrial *see also* **sārvabhauma**
bhoga	enjoyment, experience
bhoga-kalā	art for pleasure
bhraṣṭa	fallen
Brahmā	the first deity of the Hindu trinity; the Creator *see also* **Śiva, Viṣṇu**
brahmachārī	one vowed to celibacy, abstinence and religious study

brahmacharya	celibacy, religious studentship and self-restraint – this is the first of the four **āśramas**, or stages of life education
Brahman	the Supreme Spirit, the Absolute Being
brahmin	a member of the priestly caste, the highest caste of the Hindu system
Buddha	literally 'the enlightened one, the awakened one'
buddhi	intellect, reason, discrimination, judgement
buddhi-saṁyama	integration of the intelligence
chakra	wheel; circle – the **chakras** are energy centres of the body responsible for the regulation of **prāṇa** in the human system; they are situated at the points of intersection of the principal **nāḍis** or energy channels, **īda**, **piṅgalā** and **suṣumṇā**
chandra	moon
chandra-nāḍī	the channel of lunar energy *see also* **īda**
Charaka Saṁhitā	a treatise on āyurvedic medicine attributed by some to **Patañjali**
chitta	psycho-mental substitute comprising mind, intellect and ego
chittavṛtti	fluctuation of the mind; behaviour pattern, mode of being, condition or mental state; thought-wave

dāl	lentils
deśa	place
dhāraṇā	concentration or complete attention – the sixth stage of **yoga**
dharma	religion, law, merit, righteousness, good works; the essential nature of a thing; the code of conduct that sustains the soul and produces virtue, morality or religious merit – one of the four ends of human existence; that which sustains, upholds and supports
dharmendriya	organ of virtue; conscience
dhautī	one of the six **kriyās** of **haṭha-yoga**, involving the swallowing of a long piece of wet cloth to cleanse the stomach
dhyāna	meditation – the seventh stage of **yoga**
dīrgha	long
doṣa	bodily humour; fault, defect, deficiency, disease *see also* **kapha**, **pitta**, **vāta**
dveṣa	hatred, enmity, aversion
eka	one
ekāgratā	fixedness on one object or point only; close attention; focusing of the mental faculties on a single point
ekāgratā-pariṇāma	the transformation of single-pointedness; the third stage of meditation described by **Patañjali**

gārhasthya	family life – the second **āśrama**, or stage of life
ghaṭa	body; vessel
ghaṭāvasthā	understanding the body through the practice of **yoga**; stage of coming to, reaching, joining, coming in collision, exerting oneself, being intently occupied; the second stage of the practice of **yoga**
ghee	clarified butter
Goṇikā	**Patañjali**'s foster-mother
guṇa	quality – the three **guṇas** or qualities are the fundamental ingredients or constituents of nature and the cosmic substance *see also* **rajas, sattva, tamas**
guru	spiritual preceptor; teacher; one who brings light to the darkness of spiritual doubt
halāhala	the poison which emerged from the sea during the churning of the ocean by the angels and demons to release the elixir of life, and which was swallowed by **Śiva** in order that humanity might not be destroyed
halāsana	plough pose – an **āsana** in which the body, supported on the shoulders with the legs extended beyond the head and the feet touching the floor, resembles a plough

haṭha	force, will-power; forcibly, against one's will
haṭha-yoga	the way towards realisation and union of the individual with the Supreme Soul through rigorous discipline and through balancing the solar and lunar energies in the human system
Haṭha Yoga Pradīpikā	the celebrated textbook on **haṭha-yoga** written by **Svātmārāma**
īda	one of the principal **nāḍīs** or channels of energy in the body, running from the left nostril towards the base of the spine and thence to the crown of the head (also called the **chandra-nāḍī**, the channel of lunar energy) *see also* **chakra, piṅgalā, suṣumṇā**
indriya	organ, including the five organs of action and the five organs of perception *see also* **dharmendriya, jñānendriya, karmendriya**
indriya-saṁyama	integration of the organs of action and of perception
īśa	master, owner
Īśvara	the Supreme Being; God
Īśvara-praṇidhana	dedication of one's actions and one's will to God
jala	water

jala-netī	one of the six **kriyās** of **haṭha-yoga**, involving passing a thread of water from one nostril to the other
jīva	living being; creature; an individual soul, as distinguished from the universal soul
jīvámṛta	the nectar of life
jñāna	knowledge, including sacred knowledge derived from meditation on the higher truths of religion and philosophy
jñāna-mārga	the path of knowledge and understanding
jñāna-saṁyama	integration of knowledge
jñāna-yoga	the way towards realisation and union of the individual with the Supreme Soul through knowledge and understanding
jñānendriya	organ of perception; one of the five organs of hearing, touch, sight, taste and smell
Kailāsa	a mountain peak in the Himalayas, considered as the abode of **Śiva**
kaivalya	absolute freedom; perfect emancipation or detachment of the soul from matter and identification with the Supreme Spirit
Kaivalya Pada	the fourth and last chapter of **Patañjali**'s ***Yoga Sūtras***, dealing with absolute freedom
kalā	art
	see also **bhoga-kalā**, **kāma-kalā**, **yoga-kalā**

kāla	time
kāma	sensual pleasure, desire
kāma-kalā	art for the gratification of sensual desire
kapha	phlegm; one of the three humours of the body, corresponding to the element water *see also* **pitta, vāta**
kāraṇa	cause
kāraṇa-śarīra	the causal frame; the innermost of the three frames of the body, comprising the spiritual sheath of joy *see also* **śarīra**
karma	action
karma-mārga	the path of action
karma-yoga	the way towards realisation and union of the individual with the Supreme Soul through action
karmendriya	organ of action – the five **karmendriyas** are the hands, the feet and the organs of excretion, generation and speech
kevala	whole, entire, absolute, perfect, pure
kevala-kumbhaka	when the practice of **kumbhaka**, or suspension of breath between inhalation and exhalation, is so perfect that it becomes instinctive, it is known as **kevala-kumbhaka**
kleśa	pain, anguish, suffering, affliction

kośa — sheath, case; one of the five sheaths enveloping the soul: (i) **annamaya-kośa**, the anatomical sheath of nourishment corresponding to the gross anatomical body, (ii) **prāṇamaya-kośa**, the physiological sheath including the respiratory circulatory, digestive, endocrine, excretory and genital systems, (iii) **manomaya-kośa**, the psychological sheath involving awareness, feeling and judgement not derived from subjective experience, (iv) **vijñānamaya-kośa**, the intellectual sheath involving the process of reasoning and judgement derived from subjective experience, (v) **ānandamaya-kośa**, the spirit sheath of joy

see also **śarīra**

kriyā — action; cleansing process

kriyā-yoga — **yoga** of practice, **yoga** of action

Kṛṣṇa — the most celebrated hero of Hindu mythology; the eighth incarnation of **Viṣṇu**

kṣatriya — a member of the warrior caste, the second caste of the Hindu system

kumbhaka — the time of retention or suspension of breath after full inhalation or after full exhalation

see also **antara-kumbhaka, bāhya-kumbhaka, kevala-kumbhaka**

Kumbhakarṇa a gigantic demon, brother of **Rāvaṇa**, ultimately slain by **Rāma**, the hero of the ***Rāmāyana***

kuṇḍalinī coiled female serpent; the divine cosmic energy symbolised as a coiled serpent lying dormant in the mūlandhara-**chakra**, the lowest nerve centre at the base of the spinal column – this latent energy has to be aroused and made to ascend **suṣumṇā**, the main spinal channel of energy, piercing the various **chakras** right up to the sahasāra-**chakra**, the thousand-petalled lotus in the head; then the **yogī** is in union with the Supreme Universal Soul

kuṇḍalinī-yoga the way towards realisation and union of the individual with the Supreme Soul through the awakening of **kuṇḍalinī**

kūrma tortoise

Mahābhāṣya literally 'the great commentary'; **Patañjali**'s treatise on Sanskrit grammar which takes the form of a commentary on Pāṇini's Sūtras

Mahātmā high-souled, magnanimous, eminent, distinguished, mighty

manaḥ-saṁyama integration of the mind

manas the individual mind having the power and faculty of attention, selection and rejection; the ruler of the senses

manomaya-kośa the psychological sheath involving awareness, feeling and judgement not derived from subjective experience; one of the five sheaths enveloping the soul

see also **kośa, śarīra**

mantra	a sacred syllable, word, phrase or prayer which can be repeated as an aid to meditation, a formula dedicated to any particular deity, adoration addressed to a deity or deities
mārga	way, road, path *see also* **bhakti-mārga, karma-mārga, jñāna-mārga, nivṛtti-mārga, pravṛtti-mārga**
Meru	a fabulous mountain, said to be the central point of the eastern hemisphere
Mohinī	a fascinating woman, a female incarnation taken by **Viṣṇu** to beguile the demons
mokṣa	liberation; emancipation of the soul from recurring births
mokṣa-śāstra	science of liberation
mudrā	a seal; a sealing posture
nāḍī	a tubular organ of the subtle body through which flow vital, seminal and cosmic energy as well as air, water, blood, nutrients and other substances including sensations and consciousness
Naṭarāja	a name given to **Śiva** as lord of the dance (naṭa = dance; **rājā** = king)

naṭarājāsana — the **Naṭarāja** pose – in this dramatic pose the practitioner balances on one leg while bending the other leg back and stretching one arm up over the shoulder to grasp the foot behind, while the other arm is stretched forward

nidrā — sleep

nirbīja — seedless, not dependent on anything

nirbīja-samādhi — seedless state of absolute consciousness not depending on any objects, **mantras**, or other external aids

nirodha — restraint, suppression, stilling

nirodha-pariṇāma — the transformation of restraint – the first stage of meditation described by **Patañjali**, consisting of restraining the movements and fluctuations of the mind, and noting the pause or space between the restraining mind and the fluctuating mind

niṣpattyavasthā — state of completion, conclusion, termination and consummation; the fourth stage of the practice of **yoga**

nivṛtti-mārga — inward path; the way of realisation by abstaining from worldly acts and being uninfluenced by worldly desires

see also **pravṛtti-mārga**

niyama — self-purification by discipline – the second stage of **yoga**

nṛtya — dance

ojas light, splendour, lustre, energy

pada foot or leg; part of a book

padmāsana lotus pose – in this pose, the practitioner sits with the legs crossed so that each foot is placed across the opposite thigh

parichayāvasthā state of acquaintance, intimacy between body, mind and intelligence; the third stage of the practice of **yoga**

paridṛṣṭa regulated, measured

pariṇāma transformation

see also **ekāgratā-pariṇāma, nirodha-pariṇāma, samādhi-pariṇāma**

Pārvatī the consort of **Śiva**, to whom he first taught yoga

paśchimottānāsana intense posterior stretch – in this pose, the legs are stretched out along the floor and the upper body is extended forwards to lie along the top of the legs ('paśchima' literally means the west – it implies the back of the body from the head to the heels; 'uttāna' means an intense stretch)

pāta fallen

Patañjali the propounder of **yoga** philosophy, author of the ***Yoga Sūtras***, considered to be an incarnation of **Adiśeṣa**

piṅgalā one of the principal **nāḍis** or channels of energy in the body, running from the right nostril to the base of the spine and thence towards the crown of the head

	(also called the **sūrya-nāḍī,** the channel of solar energy); tawny, reddish
	see also **chakra**, **īda**, **suṣumṇā**
pitta	bile – one of the three humours of the body, corresponding to the element fire
	see also **vāta, kapha**
prāṇa	breath, respiration, wind, life force, life, vitality, energy, strength, the hidden energy in the atmospheric air
prāṇa-saṁyama	integration of breath
prāṇamaya-kośa	the physiological sheath which includes the respiratory, circulatory, digestive, endocrine, excretory and genital systems – one of the five sheaths enveloping the soul
	see also **kośa, śarīra**
prāṇāyāma	regulation of energy and life force through rhythmic control of breath – the fourth stage of **yoga**
praṇidhana	dedication, surrender
	see also **Īśvara praṇidhana**
Praśna Upaniṣad	one of the ten principal **Upaniṣads,** consisting of questions (praśna = question)
pratyāhāra	withdrawal and emancipation of the mind from the domination of the senses and sensual objects – the fifth stage of **yoga**

pravṛtti-mārga outward path; the way of action or creation

see also **nivṛtti-mārga**

pura fortress, castle, town, house, abode, body

pūraka inhalation

Purāṇa legend of the past; ancient tale of legendary or traditional history

puruṣa human soul or psychic principle; the seer; the master of the abode of the body; man

puruṣārtha aim of life in man – the four **puruṣārthas** are **dharma** (duty), **artha** (acquisition), **kāma** (pleasure) and **mokṣa** (liberation)

rāga passion, attachment to pleasure; anger

rājā king, ruler

rāja-yoga the way towards realisation and union of the individual with the Supreme Spirit by becoming the ruler of one's own mind and defeating its enemies, the chief of which are lust, anger, greed, delusion, pride and envy

rajas mobility, activity, dynamism – one of the three **guṇas** or constituents of everything which exists

see also **tamas, sattva**

Rāma the seventh incarnation of **Viṣṇu** – hero of the epic ***Rāmāyana***

Rāmakṛṣṇa Indian religious teacher (1836–86)

Rāmānuja, Śrī one of the three great **āchāryas** or preceptors of south India

Rāmāyana the celebrated epic about the exploits of **Rāma**, attributed to Valmīki

rasa taste

rasātmaka experience of various sentiments and flavours that virtuous life offers

rasātmaka-jñāna knowledge filled with the flavours of virtuous life

rasātmaka-karma action filled with the flavours of virtuousness

Rāvaṇa the demon king of Lanka (Sri Lanka) who abducted **Rāma**'s wife **Sītā** in the ***Rāmāyaṇa*** epic (**Rāvaṇa** was highly intellectual and had prodigious strength; he was an ardent devotee of **Śiva** and well versed in the **Vedas**, and is reputed to have given the accents to the **Vedic** texts so that they have remained unchanged)

rechaka exhalation; emptying of the lungs

Ṛg Veda the first of the four **Vedas** or sacred Hindu scriptures, consisting of over a thousand hymns to various deities

roga disease, illness

see also **adhibhautika-roga, adhidaivika-roga, adhyatmika-roga**

sādhana	practice; act of mastery; performance; accomplishment
Sādhana Pada	the second part of **Patañjali**'s ***Yoga Sūtras***, dealing with the means to spiritual realisation
śakti	power, energy, capacity, strength, representing the power of consciousness to act; the female aspect or consort of a divinity
sama	same, equal, even, upright
Sāma Veda	one of the four **Vedas** or sacred Hindu scriptures, consisting of metrical chants or hymns in praise of the divinities
samādhi	a state in which the aspirant is one with the object of his meditation, the Supreme Spirit governing the universe, and experiences unutterable peace and joy
Samādhi Pada	The first part of **Patañjali**'s ***Yoga Sūtras***, dealing with the state of **samādhi**
samādhi-pariṇāma	the second stage of meditation described by **Patañjali** – a state of tranquillity attained through the restraint of the fluctuations of the mind and leading towards total absorption in the greater Self
sāṁkhya	number, enumeration, calculation
saṁyama	restraint, check, control; integration: the triple phenomenon of **dhāraṇā, dhyāna** and **samādhi**

Śaṅkarāchārya, Śri Ādi one of the three great **āchāryas** or preceptors of South India

ṣaṇmukhī-mudrā a sealing posture where the apertures of the face (mouth, eyes, ears and nostrils) are closed and the mind is directed inwards to train it for meditation

sannyāsa detachment from the affairs of this world and attachment to the service of the Lord – this corresponds to the fourth **āśrama**, or stage of life

sannyāsin one who renounces worldly and family commitments to follow a spiritual path or teaching

santoṣa delight, contentment

śarīra body; frame – according to Hindu philosophy, there are three bodily frames enveloping the soul, which are further divided into five sheaths as follows: the gross or anatomical body (**sthūla-śarīra**) consists of the anatomical sheath of nourishment (**annamaya-kośa**) and is destroyed at death; the subtle body (**sūkṣma-śarīra**) comprises the physiological sheath (**prāṇamaya-kośa**), the psychological sheath (**manomaya-kośa**) and the intellectual sheath (**vijñānamaya-kośa**); the causal body (**kāraṇa-śarīra**) consists of the spiritual sheath of joy (**ānandamaya-kośa**)

see also **kośa**

śarīra-saṁyama	integration of the structural or anatomical body
sarva	all, whole
sārvabhauma	universal, pertaining to the whole world
sarvāṅgāsana	whole body pose – this is the shoulder-stand, shoulder-balance or neck-balance in which the entire body extends vertically upwards towards the feet while being supported on the shoulders
śāstra	any manual or compendium of rules, any book or treatise, especially a religious or scientific treatise, any sacred book or composition of divine authority – the word **śāstra** is normally found after the word denoting the subject of the book or is applied collectively to departments of knowledge, for example, **yoga-śāstra**, a work on **yoga** philosophy or the body of teaching on the subject of **yoga** *see also* **mokṣa-śāstra**
sattva	the illuminating, pure and good quality of everything in nature – one of the three **guṇas** or constituents of everything which exists *see also* **rajas, tamas**
satya	truth
satyam	true
śaucha	purity, cleanliness

śavāsana	corpse pose – in this **āsana** one lies on one's back like a dead body; by remaining motionless and keeping the mind still while one is fully conscious, one learns to relax, and this conscious relaxation invigorates and refreshes both body and mind – it is harder to keep the mind still than the body, so this apparently easy posture is actually one of the most difficult to master
setu-bandha-sarvāṅgāsana	bridge construction pose (setu = bridge; setu-bandha = construction of a bridge) – in this pose the body is arched and supported on the shoulders at one end and heels at the other, the arch being supported by the hands at the waist *see also* **sarvāṅgāsana**
siddha	sage, seer or prophet; semi-divine being of great purity and holiness
siddha-yoga	yoga taught by **siddhas**
Sītā	the wife of **Rāma**, heroine of the ***Rāmāyana***
Śiva	the third deity of the Hindu trinity; the Destroyer – his name means 'the auspicious one' *see also* **Brahmā, Viṣṇu**
Śiva Saṁhitā	an important **haṭha-yoga** text
śivam	auspicious
stambha	control

sthūla-śarīra	the gross body; the material or perishable body comprising the anatomical sheath which is destroyed at death – one of the three frames of the body, together with the subtle body and the causal body *see also* **śarīra**
śūdra	a member of the labourer caste, the lowest caste of the Hindu system
sūkṣma-śarīra	the subtle body – one of the three frames of the body, together with the gross body and the causal body *see also* **śarīra**
sundaram	beautiful
Sūrya	the sun god
sūrya-nāḍī	the channel of solar energy *see also* **piṅgalā**
suṣumṇā	the main **nāḍī** or channel of energy, situated inside the spinal column *see also* **chakra, ida, piṅgalā, kuṇḍalini**
sūtra	aphorism; sacred text; thread *see also* ***Yoga Sūtras***
sūtra-neti	one of the six **kriyās** of **haṭha-yoga** involving passing a thread in through one nostril and out through the other nostril or the mouth and moving it by the two ends held between the fingers
sva	self

svādhyāya self-study; education of the self by study of sacred literature

Svātmārāma author of ***Haṭha Yoga Pradīpikā***

swami a learned master; title applied to a religious teacher

tāḍāsana mountain pose – the starting point for all the standing poses, where one stands firm and erect as a mountain

tamas inertia, dormancy, darkness, ignorance – one of the three **guṇas** or constituents of everything which exists

see also **rajas, sattva**

tāṇḍavanṛtya the vigorous dance of **Śiva**, symbolising the destruction of the universe before a new cycle of creation

tapas religious fervour, burning desire to achieve a goal, scrupulousness in practice, purification, self discipline, austerity

tapasvinī a woman who has taken up religious vows; a female ascetic

tejas radiance, splendour, brilliance, light, majesty, dignity, glory

trikoṇāsana triangle pose – in this standing pose the feet are apart and the body extends to one side as one arm extends downwards and reaches the floor; a triangle is thus formed by the trunk, the arm and the leg

Upaniṣads	the philosophical portion of the **Vedas**, the most ancient sacred literature of the Hindus, dealing with the nature of man and the universe and the union of the individual soul or self with the Universal Soul – the word is derived from the prefixes 'upa' (near) and 'ni' (down) added to the root 'sad' (to sit); it means sitting down near a **guru** to receive spiritual instruction
	see also **Vedas**
vairāgya	renunciation, absence of worldly desires
vaiśya	a member of the merchant caste, the third caste of the Hindu system
vānaprastha	the third **āśrama**, or stage of life, in which one abandons family life for an ascetic life in the forest
Vasiṣṭha	a celebrated sage, author of several **Vedic** hymns
vāta	wind – one of the three humours of the body, corresponding to the element air
	see also ***kapha***, ***pitta***
Vedas	The sacred scriptures of the Hindus, classified as revealed literature and consisting of four collections called ***Ṛg-Veda*** – hymns to gods, ***Sāma Veda*** – priests' chants, ***Yajur Veda*** – sacrificial formulae in prose, and ***Atharva Veda*** – magical chants; they contain the first philosophical insights and are regarded as the final authority; each **Veda** has

	broadly two divisions, namely, **mantras** (hymns) and brāhmaṇas (precepts), the latter including āraṇyakas (liturgy) and **upaniṣads** (philosophy)
Vedic	from the **Vedas**
Vibhīṣana	the youngest brother of **Rāvaṇa**, who told the latter that his conduct in abducting **Rāma**'s wife, **Sītā**, was unrighteous and that she should be restored to her husband
vibhūti	might, power, greatness, attainment
Vibhūti Pada	the third part of the ***Yoga Sūtras*** of **Patañjali**, dealing with the powers that come to the **yogī** as a result of his spiritual practice
vid	to know; to understand
vijñāna	knowledge, wisdom, intelligence, understanding, discrimination; worldly knowledge derived from experience as opposed to knowledge of **Brahman**
vijñānamaya-kośa	the intellectual sheath involving the process of reasoning and judgement derived from subjective experience – one of the five sheaths enveloping the soul *see also* **kośa, śarīra**
viparīta	inverted, reversed, opposite, adverse, perverse, contrary
viparīta-karaṇi	a posture in which the upper body, as far as the groin, is placed as in

setu-bandha-sarvāṇgāsana, and the legs as in **sarvāṅgāsana** – this is not considered to be a complete **āsana**, but rather a form of practice (karaṇi)

Viṣṇu the second deity of the Hindu trinity; the Preserver

see also **Brahmā, Śiva**

vṛkṣa tree

vṛtti mode, modification, fluctuation

see also **chittavṛtti**

Yajur Veda one of the four **Vedas** or sacred Hindu scriptures, relating to sacrifice

yama universal moral commandments or ethical disciplines transcending creeds, countries, age and time (the five mentioned by **Patañjali** are non-violence, truth, non-stealing, continence and non-coveting) – the first stage of yoga

yoga union, communion; the union of our will to the will of God, which enables us to look evenly at life in all its aspects; the method to achieve this – the word **yoga** is derived from the root 'yuj' meaning to join, to yoke; the chief aim of **yoga** is to teach the means by which the human soul may be completely united with the Supreme Spirit pervading the universe and thus attain liberation

yoga-bhraṣṭa fallen from the grace of **yoga**

yoga-kalā	art in its highest form
Yoga Sūtras	the classical work on **yoga** by **Patañjali**, written some two thousand five hundred years ago and consisting of 196 aphorisms on **yoga**, divided into four parts dealing respectively with **samādhi**, the means by which **yoga** is attained, the powers which come to the seeker in his quest and the state of absolute liberation
yogī	one who follows the path of **yoga**
yoginī	a woman who follows the path of **yoga**

Bibliography

Books by B.K.S. Iyengar

Light on Yoga, first published by George Allen and Unwin Ltd, London 1966; paperback edition, Unwin Paperbacks, London, 1976.

The Concise Light on Yoga, Unwin Paperbacks, London 1980.

Light on Prāṇāyāma, first published by George Allen and Unwin Ltd, London 1981; paperback edition, Unwin Paperbacks 1983.

The Art of Yoga, Unwin Paperbacks, London 1985.

The above titles are all readily obtainable from bookshops in paperback editions. They can also be obtained from the Iyengar Yoga Institute, 223a Randolph Avenue, London W9 1NL, which can in addition supply *Light on Yoga* and *Light on Prāṇāyāma* in hardback editions.

Of related interest

Iyengar: His Life and Work, Timeless Books, Porthill, Idaho [1987].

Yoga: A Gem for Women, Geeta S. Iyengar, Allied Publishers Pvt. Ltd., New Delhi 1983 (This book is not readily available in the West, but can be obtained from the Iyengar Yoga Institute, 223a Randolph Avenue, London W9 1NL.)

Yoga Sūtra of Patañjali, translation and commentary, published by Shri Dharmavirsingh Mahida for Ramamani Iyengar Memorial Yoga Institute, Pune 1987 (available from the Iyengar Yoga Institute, London).

Sanskrit texts and scriptures

The following list has been compiled to help those readers who wish to make a further study of the various Sanskrit texts which have been mentioned in this book. Some of the editions listed are readily available from bookshops; others may be obtainable only through bookshops specialising in Oriental books; still others may only be obtainable through libraries. There appears to be no published translation of the *Mahābhāsya*; a Sanskrit edition has therefore been listed. Geldner's German translation of the *Ṛg Veda* and Renou's French translation of the Upaniṣads have been included on account of their excellence. Otherwise, all the books listed are English language editions.

Srīmad Bhagavadgītā, edited and translated by S.K. Belvalkar, Hindu Vishvavidyalaya, Nepal Rajya Sanskrit Series 1, Varanasi, 1959

The Bhagavad Gītā, translated and interpreted by Franklin Edgerton, Harper and Row, New York 1974 (paperback)

The Bhagavad-Gītā, translated with a commentary by R.C. Zaehner, Oxford University Press, London 1973 (paperback)

Caraka-Saṁhitā, Agniveśa's treatise refined and annotated by Caraka and redacted by Dṛḍhabala (text with English translation), edited and translated by Priyavrat Sharma, Jaikrishnadas Ayurveda Series 36, Chaukhamba Orientalia, Varanasi 1981, 83 (2 volumes)

Haṭhayogapradīpikā of Svātmārāma with the commentary Jyotsnā of Brahmānanda and English translation by Srinivas Iyangar, Adyar Library and Research Centre, Madras 1972

Haṭhayogapradīpikā of Svātmārāma, edited by Swami Digambarji and Raghunathashastri Kokaje, K.S.M.Y.M. Samiti, Lonavla 1970

The Hatha Yoga Pradipika, translated into English by Pancham Sinh,

Oriental Books Reprint Corporation, Munshiram Manoharlal Publishers Pvt. Ltd., New Delhi

The Vyākarana-Mahābhāsya of Patañjali, edited by Franz Kielhorn, revised by K. V. Abhyankar, Bandarkar Oriental Research Institute, Poona 1962–72 (3 volumes, Sanskrit only)

Ancient Indian Tradition and Mythology, translated by a board of scholars, Motilal Banarsidass, Delhi 1970– (29 volumes of translations of Purāṇas have appeared so far)

Classical Hindu Mythology: A reader in the Sanskrit Purāṇas, edited and translated by Cornelia Dimmitt and J.A.B. van Buitenen, Temple University Press, Philadelphia 1978

The Rāmāyana of Vālmīki, edited by Robert P. Goldman, Princeton University Press, Princeton 1984– (a multi-volume translation project of which 2 volumes have appeared)

The Ramayana of Valmiki, translated by Hari Prasad Shastri, Shanti Sadan, London 1952–9 (3 volumes)

Ramayana, William Buck (not a translation, but a re-telling of the Ramayana in modern English), New American Library, New York 1978 (paperback)

The Siva Samhita, translated into English by Rai Bahadur Srisa Chandra Vasu, Oriental Books Reprint Corporation, Munshiram Manoharlal Publishers Pvt. Ltd., New Delhi

The Thirteen Principal Upanishads, translated by Robert Ernest Hume, Oxford University Press, London 1971 (paperback)

The Principal Upaniṣads, edited and translated by S. Radhakrishnan, George Allen and Unwin Ltd, London 1953

Les Upanishad, text and French translation edited by Louis Renou, Adrien-Maisonneuve, Paris 1943– (The *Prasna Upaniṣad*, translated by J. Bousquet, 1948, appears in this series)

Atharvaveda-Samhitā, English translation with critical and exegetical commentary and introduction, W.D. Whitney, Harvard Oriental Series, reprint in 2 volumes, Motilal Banarsidass, Delhi 1962

The Rig Veda, an Anthology, translated by Wendy Doniger O'Flaherty, Penguin, Harmondsworth 1981

Der Rig-Veda, German translation by K.F. Geldner, Harvard Oriental Series, volumes 33–5, Cambridge 1951 (index, volume 4 by J. Nobel, 1957)

The Hymns of the Sāmaveda, translated by R.T.H. Griffith, E.J. Lazarus, Benares 1963

The Veda of the Black Yajus School entitled Taittirīya Saṃhitā, Arthur Berriedale Keith, Motilal Banarsidass, Delhi 1967 (2 volumes)

The Texts of the White Yajurveda, translated by R.T.H. Griffith, Varanasi 1899

The Yoga-System of Patañjali, James Haughton Woods, Harvard Oriental Series, volume 17, Cambridge 1914

Patañjali's Yoga Sutras with the commentary of Vyāsa and the gloss of Vāchaspati Misra, translated by Rāma Prasāda with an introduction by Rai Bahadur Srisa Chandra Vasu, Oriental Books Reprint Corporation, Munshiram Manoharlal Pvt. Ltd., New Delhi 1978

The Yoga Aphorisms of Patañjali, translated by Shri Purohit Swami with an introduction by W.B. Yeats, Faber and Faber, London 1987

Index